# 40 DAYS TO
# BETTER
# LIVING

## DIABETES

BARBOUR
PUBLISHING

Published by Barbour Publishing, Inc., P.O. Box 719, Uhrichsville,
Ohio 44683 www.barbourbooks.com

*Our mission is to publish and distribute inspirational products
offering exceptional value and biblical encouragement to the
masses.*

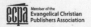
Member of the
Evangelical Christian
Publishers Association

Printed in the United States of America.

# TABLE OF CONTENTS

# Welcome,
# from Dr. Scott Morris,
# Founder of the Church Health Center

I first came to Memphis in 1986. I had no personal ties to Memphis and did not know anyone here. Having completed theological and medical education, I was determined to begin a health care ministry for the working poor. The next year, the doors of the Church Health Center opened with one doctor—me—and one nurse. We saw twelve patients the first day. Today we handle about 36,000 patient visits a year and 120,000 visits to our Wellness facility. A staff of 250 people shares a ministry of healing and wellness while hundreds more volunteer time and services.

So what sets us apart from other community clinics around the country?

The Church Health Center is fundamentally about the Church. We care for our patients without relying on government funds because God calls the Church to healing work. Jesus' life was about healing the whole person—body and spirit—and the Church is Jesus in the world. His message is our message. His ministry is our ministry. Local congregations embrace this calling and help make our work possible.

More than two decades of caring for the working uninsured makes one thing plain: health care needs to change. In the years that the Church Health Center has cared for people in Memphis, we've seen that two-thirds of our patients seek treatment for illness that healthier living can prevent or control. We realize that if we want to make a lasting difference in our patients' lives, the most effective strategy is encouraging overall wellness in body and spirit. At a fundamental level, we must transform what the words *well* and *health* mean in the minds of most people.

To do that, we developed the Model for Healthy Living. Living healthy lives doesn't just mean that you see the doctor regularly. Rather, healthy living means that all aspects of your life are in balance. Your faith, work, nutrition, movement, family and friends, emotions, and medical health all contribute to a life filled with more joy, more love, and more connection to God.

## How to Use This Book

This book gives you the chance to improve your health in whatever way is needed for managing your diabetes. For the next forty days, we invite you to be inspired by the real-life people whose lives have been changed by the Church Health Center. Each day gives us a new chance to more effectively manage our diabetes, so each day we will give you helpful ways that you can make your life a healthier one.

Some days you may choose to focus on just one or two of our "tips": Faith Life, Medical, Movement, Work, Emotional, Family and Friends, or Nutrition. Some days you may want to try all of them. The important thing is to remember that God calls us to an abundant life, and we can always make changes to strive for better health as it relates to our diabetes.

Forty days and numerous ways to live a healthy life—come and join us on the journey!

# Week 1

## Michael's Story

When Michael started coming to the Church Health Center in 2003, he knew that he had diabetes, but he knew very little about how to manage his illness. He felt ill most of the time because he was often tired and sick. His work suffered, and he worried that he might actually lose his job. His solution to feeling ill was adding more and more insulin and medication to his regimen rather than really changing his lifestyle.

Then a friend recommended he look into the Church Health Center. At first he was skeptical, thinking that he couldn't exercise because he felt too ill. When he started coming to the Church Health Center, he met with a nutritionist and a wellness expert who helped him develop strategies for managing his illness and medication.

He started walking every day, and he took cooking classes to help him learn how to prepare diabetic-friendly meals. Before too long, he was managing his disease with more confidence than he ever had in his life.

Now, at the age of sixty-two, Michael says that he feels healthier than ever. He no longer takes insulin and manages his diabetes with diet, exercise, and a couple medications. "When I started, I didn't know how good I could feel," he says. "I am so thankful for my health now. I didn't even think it was possible."

# Day 1:
## New Beginnings

---

## Morning Reflection

Congratulations! Today we are setting foot on a journey to better manage diabetes. It is a journey that will take us on highs and lows and will lead us toward a wellness-oriented lifestyle. Diabetes can be a difficult diagnosis to live with, and even though it is a manageable disease, it can be intimidating. But each journey has a beginning, and today is yours! Starting today, we will focus on taking those first steps toward diabetes management and healthy living.

### Faith Life
If you do not have a journal, start one today. Take a few minutes and write ten words that describe your faith life right now. Be honest and include both positive and negative aspects of your faith life.

### Medical
Make a list of your medical concerns. Diabetes is among them, but other medical issues often accompany diabetes. Having a list of your medical concerns will help you to set goals and measure your progress.

### Movement
We all have to start somewhere. Go for a walk today, walking as far as you can. Do not exhaust yourself, and stop when you feel you need to. Make a note in a journal so that you can track your progress.

### Work
Today take a few minutes and write in your journal about what makes up your "work." Keep in mind that work can mean your job, volunteering, and parenting. As we move forward on the journey, it will be very important to find ways to make our work healthy.

### Emotional
Our emotional wellness is an important part of overall wellness, and an aspect that often gets overlooked. Today write in your journal about your feelings as you begin the journey. Are you excited? Frightened? Anxious?

### Family and Friends
The journey toward wellness is not one that you can take in isolation. Support from family and friends is very important. Today write the names of your family and friends who will support you on this journey to diabetes management.

### Nutrition
Do you have a food journal? If you do not, start one today or add a daily food log to your current journal. Having a place to keep track of what you eat will help as you work to form better health habits.

## Evening Wrap-up

*In the beginning God created the heavens and the earth. Now the earth was formless and empty, darkness was over the surface of the deep, and the Spirit of God was hovering over the waters.*
GENESIS 1:1–2

We all need to begin somewhere. In fact, even God talks about beginnings. We all have heard the phrase "In the beginning. . ." When we look at this passage from Genesis, we see that the earth was "formless and empty." We are beginning our journey toward diabetes management, and it might feel like the road ahead is "formless and empty." After all, the road ahead is somewhat of a mystery. But we can move forward knowing that God walks with us, offering us strength and encouragement along the way.

*God of Creation, I know that You made me from nothing. Help me today to know that I do not walk this journey alone. In Your holy name, Amen.*

# Day 2:
## Foundations

## Morning Reflection

Before we build a house, we must build the foundation. The foundation offers support for the roof and walls and bears the load for everything else that is to come. Wellness and diabetes management are lifelong processes that are never truly complete. But on our six-week journey, we will lay the foundation for the longer road ahead. So today we will turn our focus to laying the groundwork that will bear the load of the changes to come.

### Faith Life
Foundation is a word that occasionally comes up in discussions of faith and spirituality. Today take five minutes and write about the foundation of your faith life right now.

### Medical
Laying a good medical foundation is very important for the journey to managing diabetes. Today make a list of the things that you are doing now to manage your diabetes.

### Movement
After you take a shower, move your body around a bit and spend five to ten minutes doing some light stretching. Bend and touch your toes and reach your

arms across your chest. If it hurts, pull back on the stretch a bit.

## Work
Sometimes our lack of wellness can keep us from doing the kind of work that we want to do. Take five minutes and write about a time that you found yourself unable to do the work you wanted to do. Keep in mind that work can be your career, but it does not have to be.

## Emotional
Deep breathing can help you get centered, release stress, and energize yourself. Take five minutes today and practice breathing. Close your eyes, breathe in through your nose and out through your mouth.

## Family and Friends
Family dinners are a wonderful way to connect with your family and friends. They are also a wonderful time to try new recipes. Today schedule a family dinner for sometime in the next week.

## Nutrition
If you have not spoken to a nutritionist, set up an appointment today. A nutritionist can help you create a diet that is specific to your particular needs and can help you control your diabetes.

## Evening Wrap-up

*"In the beginning, Lord, you laid the foundations
of the earth, and the heavens are the work of your
hands. They will perish, but you remain; they will
all wear out like a garment. You will roll them up
like a robe; like a garment they will be changed.
But you remain the same, and
your years will never end."*
HEBREWS 1:10–12

As we move forward, we need to have a solid
foundation upon which to build. But as we strive
to make our own foundation, we may need to be
reminded that it is God, who "laid the foundations
of the earth," who will continue even after those
foundations have worn.

*Loving God, I know that You will persist long after
the mountains have crumbled. Remind me today that
You are my foundation, even when everything else
might be shifting. In Your holy name, Amen.*

# Day 3:
## Motivation

## Morning Reflection

As we set out on this path toward wellness and diabetes management, we are all taking these first steps for different reasons. Part of our motivation may be simply wanting to feel better. More often, however, our motivation goes beyond the desire to be healthy. Maybe we want to be able to play more with our kids. Maybe we want to stop taking so many medications. Whatever our motivation, it is important to know it and remember it as we set out on the journey, because this motivation will keep us going when the road gets difficult.

Faith Life
Take five minutes and write in your journal about your spiritual motivation for being on this wellness journey. Where is God for you on this journey? Is He with you?

Medical
Write down your medical motivation. Try to be as specific as possible. For example, if you take medications that you would like to wean yourself off of, write down the specific medications. Remember that this may or may not be possible, depending

on your doctor's recommendations, but identifying your medical goals will help you stay motivated.

## Movement
Make sure when you begin a walking program that you check your blood sugar. Exercise can lower your blood sugar, so make sure you have something with you, like glucose gel, to help quickly raise your blood sugar if it drops too low.

## Work
Sometimes our work can provide the motivation we need to begin the journey toward wellness. Today take five minutes and write about ways that your work can motivate you.

## Emotional
Today take five minutes and write about your emotional motivation. Try to be honest, and be as specific as possible. Why are you setting out on this journey now?

## Family and Friends
Our family and friends can be particularly powerful motivation on the journey toward wellness. Today think of two people in your life who can help motivate you when the going gets tough.

## Nutrition

Most of us have a standard grocery list. What is yours? Take a few minutes today and write up a standard list of the food that you generally buy in a week, and then ask if you think this list is diabetic friendly.

## Evening Wrap-up

*Then God said, "Let us make mankind in our
image, in our likeness, so that they may rule over
the fish in the sea and the birds in the sky, over
the livestock and all the wild animals, and over
all the creatures that move along the ground."
So God created mankind in his own image,
in the image of God he created them;
male and female he created them.*
GENESIS 1:26–27

We are all created in God's image. That is, our very
bodies bear the image of our Creator. But for many of
us, it is difficult to love our bodies as God does. After
all, God cares for and loves all of creation. Part of this
journey to wellness is learning to see ourselves as
God sees us. God loves creation, and God loves us.

*Loving God, I know that You have created me in Your
image. Help me to remember that You care for me as I
move forward on this journey. In Your holy name, Amen.*

# Day 4:
## Expectations

## Morning Reflection

Every time we set out on a journey, we have expectations for that road. Having expectations is simply a part of life. But on the road to wellness, we can set up expectations for ourselves and for others that are either realistic or unrealistic. When we have unrealistic expectations, we can get in our own way. Our own expectations can (and do) shape our day-to-day experience of wellness and faith. So today we will focus on realistic expectations.

Faith Life
We all have expectations of God in our lives. What are your expectations of God on this journey? Take five minutes today and write about your expectations of God.

Medical
Our expectations are often shaped by previous experiences. What are your expectations for the medical professionals in your life? The next time you have a doctor's appointment, discuss your expectations with him or her.

## Movement
Spend ten minutes stretching today. Can you stretch any farther than you did a couple of days ago? What are your expectations for a couple of days from now?

## Work
When you take a break at work, what do you usually do? Take a trip to a vending machine? Grab a cup of coffee? Today try going for a short walk instead of eating during your break.

## Emotional
If we have unrealistic expectations for ourselves, then our stress level will increase rather than become more manageable. Take five minutes and write, as honestly as you can, what your expectations are for the next six weeks, whether they are realistic or not.

## Family and Friends
Sometimes we can feel that our family and friends have particular expectations of us, and that can add to stress that we are already feeling. Today talk to a friend or family member about your journey and what your expectations include.

## Nutrition
Our nutritional habits will not change overnight. Nor will our tastes. Today make a list of your favorite foods. Are they healthy foods? Comfort foods? Over the next six weeks, work on finding more nutritional ways to enjoy your favorite foods.

## Evening Wrap-up

*But do not forget this one thing, dear friends:*
*With the Lord a day is like a thousand years,*
*and a thousand years are like a day.*
*The Lord is not slow in keeping his promise,*
*as some understand slowness.*
*Instead he is patient with you, not wanting anyone*
*to perish, but everyone to come to repentance.*
2 Peter 3:8–9

We all have expectations of ourselves and of God. Expectations are simply a part of life. But as Peter reminds us, our expectations do not always match reality. God, however, is faithful, and we can rest assured that He walks this journey with us, even when we don't quite notice it. God's love is stronger than any expectations we might have for ourselves.

*God of faithfulness, I know that even when my expectations do not match reality, You walk with me. Help me to see Your love, and care for me as I continue on this journey.*
*In Your holy name, Amen.*

# Day 5:
## Setbacks

---

## Morning Reflection

On this journey, there will be times when we will feel unstoppable. Everything will be going well and according to plan, and then something will happen. Setbacks will and do happen. Making true progress on the journey to wellness and diabetes management involves moving forward and then dealing with setbacks. True progress is slow, measured over a long period of time. Setbacks, when we have them, can provide us an excuse to give up, but they can also provide us an opportunity for growth.

Faith Life
Think of a time in your faith life when you experienced a setback. Spend five minutes writing about that time. How did you move past it? Did you talk to a friend? Your pastor? Did you spend more time reading the Bible and praying?

Medical
Medical setbacks (such as a diabetes diagnosis) can be devastating. But such hurdles need not be the end of the world, nor should they be cause to give up. Today write out a plan for dealing with medical setbacks to discuss when you next meet with your doctor.

## Movement
Walk around your home taking two steps forward and then one step backward. Notice how you still make forward progress, even when every third step is a step back.

## Work
Work is a place where many of us have setbacks. Stress and time constraints make it easy to fall into old (and bad) habits such as vending machine lunches and caffeinated, sugary sodas. Today try bringing a stress ball or some Silly Putty to your workplace to relieve stress.

## Emotional
Many of us are "programmed" to assign more value to our failures than to our successes. Today make a list of successes or small victories that you had today. For example, "I drank water instead of soda with my lunch." Celebrate those successes!

## Family and Friends
When you stumble, your family and friends can help to remind you of your successes. Today name two people whom you can count on to offer encouragement and perspective in the event of a setback.

## Nutrition
Nutritional setbacks happen. We have an occasional doughnut or eat a little more than we had intended at a dinner out. Though the temptation is to starve

ourselves the next day, the better way to deal with those setbacks is to simply get back to healthy, moderate eating the next day.

## Evening Wrap-up

*When times are good, be happy;*
*but when times are bad, consider this:*
*God has made the one as well as the other.*
ECCLESIASTES 7:14

This journey, just like every excursion, will be full of ups and downs. It will be full of mountains and molehills, good days and bad. If we expect every day to be a complete success, then we are likely to feel let down or discouraged. Remember that God is with us through all our highs and lows. The author of Ecclesiastes reminds us that there are good times and bad, and that we can celebrate the good times, even while being comforted in the bad times.

*God of the journey, thank You for making all days,*
*good and bad. Help me today and in the days ahead*
*to remember that You have made all of my days.*
*In Your holy name, Amen.*

# Day 6:
# Setting Goals

## Morning Reflection

This journey toward wellness and diabetes management is about making changes, both in the short term and in the long term. But if we make changes without a sense of where we are headed, we may end up feeling overwhelmed or frantic. Setting realistic goals is very important to making lifestyle changes. In particular, effective goal setting can help us stay focused at times when we meet barriers, and when we are the closest to giving up. Today we will work on setting healthy short-term and long-term goals for the journey.

### Faith Life

Take five minutes today and write down one practical and concrete goal for the next six weeks. For example, set a goal that you will pray once a day each day at a particular time. The more specific and concrete the goal, the easier it will be to achieve it.

### Medical

Weight loss is often a medical goal set by people who are trying to better manage their diabetes. If this is your goal, try to aim for one to two pounds per week. While weight loss can certainly be a part of a wellness-oriented lifestyle, it is not healthy to lose weight too rapidly.

## Movement
Today write down three goals related to exercise and place those goals in a place where you will see them often. (For example: Walk for ten minutes without taking a break. Do ten wall push-ups. Do ten sit-ups.)

## Work
Make a copy of your movement and nutritional goals to take to work. Remember that wellness is not confined to the home. Having a copy of your wellness goals at work will help you to stay focused when you are away from home.

## Emotional
Diabetes can be exacerbated by stress. Today write down a specific and concrete goal for managing your stress. Remember to set a definitive time frame for your goal.

## Family and Friends
Are you embarking on this journey on your own or with a friend or some family members? Having a companion can be very helpful. Think today about a friend or family member to whom you might reach out.

## Nutrition
What would you like to change about your nutritional habits? Eat less fat? More vegetables? Better portion sizes? Write down five nutritional goals for the next six weeks.

## Evening Wrap-up

*Train yourself to be godly. For physical training
is of some value, but godliness has value for all
things, holding promise for both the present life
and the life to come. This is a trustworthy saying
that deserves full acceptance. That is why we labor
and strive, because we have put our hope in the
living God, who is the Savior of all people,
and especially of those who believe.*
1 TIMOTHY 4:7–10

We are now setting out on a journey of physical and
spiritual training. Wellness and diabetes management
are about our bodies and our spirits. When we
neglect one in favor of the other, we forget that God
created us as body and spirit. Paul reminds us in his
first letter to Timothy that our hope in God can offer
us encouragement and purpose as we strive toward
our goal.

*Loving God, I have put my hope in You.
I pray today that You will offer me the encouragement
I need as I continue on this journey.
In Your holy name, Amen.*

# Day 7:
## Celebrate

## Morning Reflection

Congratulations! We have completed the first week of our journey! At this point, we can take a step back and reflect on everything that we have accomplished this week. Maybe you are not used to celebrating our own accomplishments, but celebration is an important part of the journey. As we move forward, we can take time to celebrate even the small victories. So today we will focus on ways that we can celebrate.

### Faith Life
Faith is an important part of wellness, but wellness is also important to faith. Keep in mind that God entered this world as a person with a body. Go for a walk today, and pray as you walk for God to be present in your body as well as your spirit.

### Medical
Do you remember how to check your pulse? Try again today to calculate your resting heart rate. Knowing your numbers will help you track your improvement throughout the next five weeks.

## Movement

Spend ten minutes doing some jumping jacks or another vigorous activity that might raise your heart rate. Try to make it an activity that you enjoy.

## Work

As you sit at your desk at work, take a few minutes each hour and stand up. Do some squats or lunges to elevate your heart rate and strengthen your legs. This will give you a boost in energy and will allow you some exercise during the day.

## Emotional

On the journey to wellness, it is important to periodically reward yourself. But it is common for us to reward ourselves with food. Today make a list of rewards for yourself that are not food related.

## Family and Friends

Schedule a small celebration with your family and friends. Make a healthy meal at home, and bring your friends and family into the kitchen to share what you are learning on your journey.

## Nutrition

Make a grocery list today that looks forward. Be sure to include lots of vegetables (fresh or frozen, or low-sodium canned), whole grains, and lean protein.

# Evening Wrap-up

*Sing to the L&#820;ORD a new song; sing to the L&#820;ORD,*
*all the earth. Sing to the L&#820;ORD, praise his*
*name; proclaim his salvation day after day.*
*Declare his glory among the nations,*
*his marvelous deeds among all peoples.*
*For great is the L&#820;ORD and most worthy of praise.*
P&#820;SALM 96:1–4

Diabetes management is not an easy task, which is why it is important to celebrate along the way. When we celebrate, we remember that God walks this journey with us and celebrates our successes with us. As we remember our triumphs, we also praise God who created us and loves us.

*God of joy, You are great and worthy of praise. I pray today that You would help me as I reflect on my week to celebrate even those small successes that put me on the path toward wellness and diabetes management.*
*In Your holy name, Amen.*

# Week 2

## Sally's Story

Sally loved to eat butter. She loved to cook, and butter was always one of her favorite and most important ingredients. Then one day, when she was forty-six years old, she got some bad news from her doctor. "I had diabetes and high blood pressure." Her doctor told her in no uncertain terms that it was time to change her lifestyle.

"I was devastated," Sally said. "I loved to cook for my family and church and friends. I felt like my life was over."

But Sally's doctor recommended that she look to the Church Health Center for guidance. She took a class on diabetes management and started an exercise program. She started walking every day. Then one day she signed up for a cooking class. "I thought I would hate it because I just knew the food would be bland and boring." But much to her surprise, Sally found that she could love cooking this new way, and the food was anything but boring. "I never realized that food could be so colorful!" she said.

Today Sally is managing her diabetes with diet and exercise, and her blood pressure is within a normal range. And she still loves to cook for her family, her friends, and her church.

# Day 8:
## Habits

## Morning Reflection

Diabetes management and wellness are largely about habits. They are both about habits that we have and about habits that we want to form. Diabetes management, in short, is about changing habits. Habits can be very difficult to change because they are often so deeply ingrained in our day-to-day living that we do not even realize what we are doing. Today we will turn our focus to understanding what our habits are and forming strategies to change them.

### Faith Life
Habits do not have to be bad habits. Today make a list of your faith habits. For example, praying before meals or reading the Bible in the morning.

### Medical
Are you in the habit of recording your blood glucose levels? Monitoring your blood glucose can help you and your doctor decide on the most effective mode of treatment for you. Check your levels before meals, two hours after meals, and before bedtime. Record your levels in your journal.

## Movement
Many of us do not move enough out of sheer habit. Today go for a walk either after lunch or dinner to give your metabolism a little boost after your meal.

## Work
What do you usually do when you get home after work? Do you watch television? Cook dinner? Today take ten minutes or so to stretch or walk before you start your usual "after-work" routine.

## Emotional
Emotions are highly habitual. We can get into the habit of always feeling "busy" or "overwhelmed" or "stressed." Today practice smiling twenty-five times. Just the act of smiling will trick your brain into feeling differently.

## Family and Friends
We have collective habits as well as individual habits. Today think about the last time you were together with your family. Write about that time. Did you eat? Play games? Argue? What are your collective habits?

## Nutrition
Most of us have formed rather poor nutritional habits, including drinking soda. Don't drink your calories today. Substitute water or unsweetened iced tea for sugary soda. (Hint: even diet soda contains sodium and other ingredients that are not good for you.)

## Evening Wrap-up

*Therefore, I urge you, brothers and sisters,*
*in view of God's mercy, to offer your bodies as a*
*living sacrifice, holy and pleasing to God—this is*
*your true and proper worship. Do not conform to*
*the pattern of this world, but be transformed by*
*the renewing of your mind. Then you will be*
*able to test and approve what God's will is—*
*his good, pleasing and perfect will.*
ROMANS 12:1–2

Our habits are persistent and tough, and in order to change those habits, we must be persistent and tough. It can be difficult, even to the point of feeling that it's impossible to make real and lasting changes to our habits. But we also know that God walks the journey with us, offering us strength and encouragement as we work to be transformed and renewed.

*Loving God, help me to see my habits today and give me*
*the strength and encouragement to change them and*
*become transformed on this journey to diabetes*
*management. In Your holy name, Amen.*

# Day 9:
## Triggers

## Morning Reflection

Our habits do not work alone. Even when we do not realize it, we may have emotional and behavioral triggers that set into motion habits and behaviors that we may or may not actually be aware of. One way that we can help gain control over those habits is to be aware of the triggers that throw us into them. So today we will work to identify some of our triggers.

### Faith Life
Quiet meditation or "centering" is a wonderful tool to use in faith life. Today sit for five minutes and concentrate on being quiet. Try to quiet your "inner voice" and find peace with being still.

### Medical
Do you know the signs of low blood sugar (hypoglycemia)? They include feeling shaky, fast heartbeat, sweating, dizziness, anxiety, hunger, blurry vision, weakness or fatigue, and headache. However, hypoglycemia does not always come with symptoms. The only way to know for sure is to have an accurate glucose reading.

### Movement
Today each time you yawn during the day, do five jumping jacks. This will help to give you a boost of

energy when you are feeling tired and will give you a chance to try a new "trigger."

## Work
Today try to identify your work triggers. For example, do you grab a cup of coffee or a soda every time you walk past the break room? Try keeping some herbal tea at your desk instead. This will help you to stay hydrated and avoid becoming overcaffeinated.

## Emotional
Emotional triggers are very strong and often difficult to detect. Today take some time and write in your journal about what you do when you feel happy, bored, and sad. Knowing our reactions to these emotions can help us to avoid unhealthy reactions when we have them.

## Family and Friends
Family and friends provide us with some of our most pronounced triggers because families can easily fall into patterns of behavior that are largely out of our control. The next time you have a family gathering, try to focus on the fellowship and enjoyment rather than on food.

## Nutrition
Consistency with your carbohydrate intake at each meal throughout your day will help to stabilize your glucose levels. An average-sized, active man should get 60–75 grams of carbohydrates per meal. An average-sized woman should get 45–60 grams.

## Evening Wrap-up

*"Why spend money on what is not bread,
and your labor on what does not satisfy?
Listen, listen to me, and eat what is good,
and you will delight in the richest of fare.
Give ear and come to me; listen,
that you may live."*
Isaiah 55:2–3

The journey toward wellness and diabetes management is, in many ways, about learning how to feed ourselves. We feed ourselves in every aspect of our lives, and God wants us to choose those things that will nourish us. Isaiah reminds us of this when he says, "Why spend money on what is not bread?" When we allow triggers to control our behaviors, we may not be getting the nourishment that we need. As we move forward on this journey, we will learn how to nourish ourselves better.

*Loving God, help me to recognize what will surely satisfy
and what will not. Help me to make choices for
nourishment. In Your holy name, Amen.*

# Day 10:
## Cleaning House

## Morning Reflection

Sometimes when we make changes in our lives, we need to take the time to clean—to clean our houses, our bodies, and even our spirits. The process of cleaning helps us to get out the old and make room for the new. In our journey toward diabetes management, cleaning house can allow us a new beginning. Cleaning our pantries, our bedrooms, and our offices can help us to move forward on the journey toward wellness.

### Faith Life
Today try again to sit quietly, meditating and centering yourself. Clear away the clutter of your mind, and turn your focus to your breathing. Breathe in and let God in.

### Medical
When was the last time you cleaned out your medicine cabinet? Lots of accidents can be avoided by disposing of expired and old medication. Today take inventory of your medicine cabinet and throw out anything expired or unusable.

### Movement
Take a half hour today and do some chores around the house. Vacuuming, mopping, dusting, and cleaning

countertops can raise your heart rate. As an added bonus, when you're done, you will enjoy a clean house!

## Work
Clear some space at work (in your desk or another convenient space) where you can store some healthy snacks: unsalted nuts or dried fruit. Then when you have a break, instead of going to the vending machine, reach for your healthy snacks and take a walk around the office.

## Emotional
To calm some of the clutter in your mind today, set aside some time to have a hot bath. As you soak, focus on breathing in and out, and let your body relax.

## Family and Friends
Recruit some of your family and friends to clean your kitchen, and especially your pantry today. Take the opportunity to throw out expired foods, as well as highly processed foods that are high in sodium, sugar, or fat.

## Nutrition
Do not be a member of the "Clean Plate Club." Today pay attention to your feelings of hunger as you eat. Let your hunger, rather than your plate, dictate how much you eat.

## Evening Wrap-up

*That, however, is not the way of life you learned when you heard about Christ. . . . You were taught, with regard to your former way of life, to put off your old self. . .to be made new in the attitude of your minds; and to put on the new self, created to be like God in true righteousness and holiness.*
EPHESIANS 4:20–24

Each day we have the opportuninty to begin again. There will be days when we need to stop, take stock, and make room. Cleaning can give us space to change course if necessary. Though it may be difficult, Paul reminds us that we can "put off" former habits, our "old selves," to make room for Christ. Likewise we can clear the way for new progress on the journey.

*Loving God, I know that You can make all things new, including me. Help me today as I make room for the new while I clean out the old. In Your holy name, Amen.*

# Day 11:
## Attitude

## Morning Reflection

In this journey toward wellness and diabetes management, our progress will depend on many factors. One of the most important, however, is the attitude that we bring to the journey. A positive attitude can keep us motivated and moving forward even when things are not going the way we want them to go. A negative attitude can hold us back even when things are going well. Today we will focus on strategies for keeping a positive attitude.

<u>Faith Life</u>
Take a short walk today. While you walk, pray that God will give you encouragement to continue on this journey. When you finish your walk, have a glass of water, and remember that God has provided that water for you.

<u>Medical</u>
Remember that medications can have side effects— some are physical and some are emotional. If you are having emotional side effects (such as depression, anxiety, euphoria) or physical side effects, let your doctor know as soon as possible.

## Movement
Many of us eat when we feel bored or overwhelmed. Today if you feel bored (but are not actually hungry), instead of snacking, try doing some simple stretches, such as neck rolls and arm crosses.

## Work
If you are having a difficult day at work, make a plan to do something you enjoy when the day is done (cook a delicious dinner, go for a walk outside, etc.). Write your plan on a note card that you can leave in a visible place.

## Emotional
When you are tired and sleep deprived, having a positive attitude becomes even more difficult than it might normally be. Tonight try to go to bed at a reasonable hour, allowing seven to eight hours for sleep.

## Family and Friends
Your family and friends can be a wonderful source of encouragement when you are feeling discouraged. Today make a list of five friends or family members who will help you at times when you need some encouragement.

## Nutrition
Choosing whole-grain carbohydrates, such as whole-wheat bagels, English muffins, or toast can help you control your blood glucose better than biscuits, doughnuts, or muffins. Today choose whole grains over simple carbohydrates.

## Evening Wrap-up

*"Here is my servant, whom I uphold,*
*my chosen one in whom I delight; I will put my*
*Spirit on him, and he will bring justice to the*
*nations. . . . A bruised reed he will not break,*
*and a smoldering wick he will not snuff out.*
*In faithfulness he will bring forth justice;*
*he will not falter or be discouraged till he*
*establishes justice on earth. In his teaching*
*the islands will put their hope."*
ISAIAH 42:1, 3–4

On this journey, it will become increasingly important to find ways to maintain a positive attitude. Discouragement happens, but with a positive attitude, we can find ways to move forward in spite of it. In this passage from Isaiah, we are reminded that God is faithful, and that God offers us hope even when we cannot see it for ourselves.

*Loving God, help me to hold on to hope as I continue on this journey. Help me keep a positive attitude today and all days. In Your holy name, Amen.*

# Day 12:
## Wholeness

## Morning Reflection

When we have a wellness-oriented goal, such as weight loss or diabetes management, our focus often turns to one particular aspect of wellness. But the danger in that kind of focus is that we can lose sight of our whole body and see our entire selves as only one part—a heart, stomach, a mouth. We are, however, whole beings made of body and spirit. Our wellness is about wholeness. So today we will turn our focus to seeing ourselves as whole beings.

### Faith Life

Take five minutes today to pray. While you pray, wiggle your fingers and your toes. Sit down and stand up. Take a deep breath in and let it out. Think about how your entire body can pray, rather than just your spirit.

### Medical

Do you know the basic facts about your diabetes pills? Today write down the names of your medications, your dosage (how much you need to take), and when you need to take it. Place the fact sheet on your refrigerator or in another easy-to-find space.

## Movement

Today put on some music and spend some time dancing. Do not worry about looking silly. Feel your body move—your head, your back, your legs. Have fun as you feel your body working as a whole unit together.

## Work

Most of us work using one aspect of our personality more than other parts. Today try to take five minutes at work and use another aspect of your body or personality. If you sit at a computer all day, go for a short walk. If you're on the phone, take a moment to stretch, and if you stand all day, find a quiet place to sit.

## Emotional

If you start feeling pulled in seventeen different directions today, pull yourself together by taking a hot shower. The water can drown out some of the noise of your life, and when you are finished, you will feel a little more "whole."

## Family and Friends

Today make a list of the different ways that your friends care for you. Has anyone ever brought you soup when you were sick? Do you have someone you can call when you are feeling down? Realize that your friends care for your whole self.

## Nutrition

When you have a meal in a restaurant, watch out for words like sweet and sour, honey glazed, or honey mustard. These sauces often contain quite a bit of sugar.

## Evening Wrap-up

*Now no shrub had yet appeared on the earth and
no plant had yet sprung up. . .but streams came up
from the earth and watered the whole surface of
the ground. Then the L*ORD *God formed a man
from the dust of the ground and breathed
into his nostrils the breath of life,
and the man became a living being.*
G*ENESIS* 2:5–7

We do not look at God's creation and see only the
leaf of a tree or the sun shining through the clouds.
Instead, when we speak of God's creation, we tend
to speak of the whole of creation. So, too, when
we speak of wellness, we must consider our whole
selves, body and spirit. We can keep in mind that
God created us body and spirit.

*Loving God, You have breathed the breath of life into me.
I pray that You would help me see the wonder and
wholeness of Your creation in myself.
In Your holy name, Amen.*

# Day 13:
## Enjoyment

## Morning Reflection

Many times when we talk about healthy living, we are talking about depriving ourselves of the things (especially food) that we enjoy. But the journey toward wellness is about living well and living with abundance, not deprivation. On the path to diabetes management, it is true that some foods will need to be passed over in favor of other healthier options. But we will (hopefully) find that in managing our diabetes and living wellness-oriented lives, we can enjoy living more than we did before.

### Faith Life
While our faith life is important, it does not need to be devoid of enjoyment. Today when you find your-self laughing or smiling, say a prayer of thanks.

### Medical
The next time you have an appointment with your primary care provider, talk to him or her about whether you should see a podiatrist or a physical therapist. Both of these specialists can help you care for your feet, which can be necessary with diabetes management.

## Movement
Try not to look at exercise as a chore. Instead seek to find ways to exercise that you enjoy. Go for a walk around your neighborhood or play a game of basketball. The more you enjoy exercise, the more you will do it.

## Work
While work is not often considered fun, it helps to find aspects of your work that you enjoy. Today make a list of some things that you enjoy about your work, even if it is as simple as liking the people with whom you work.

## Emotional
If we do not spend time enjoying ourselves, we can easily become overwhelmed. Today spend at least ten minutes doing something you truly enjoy. Try to take time each day to do something you appreciate.

## Family and Friends
Our family and friends can really help us find enjoyment when we are feeling overwhelmed. Today schedule an evening out with some friends and family. Go to a healthy restaurant and try something on the menu that you may not have had otherwise.

## Nutrition
Keep in mind that alcohol can make your blood sugar dip too low. It can also interfere with some forms of diabetes medication. If drinking alcohol is a regular part of your lifestyle, talk with your health-care team about how best to enjoy it safely.

# Evening Wrap-up

*I will praise you with the harp for your faithfulness, my God; I will sing praise to you with the lyre, Holy One of Israel. My lips will shout for joy when I sing praise to you—I whom you have delivered. My tongue will tell of your righteous acts all day long.*
PSALM 71:22–24

We are created for life, and for praise and joy. Living a wellness-oriented lifestyle should not hinder that joy but should help us to enjoy life more. Though healthy living is often stereotyped as depriving ourselves of enjoyment, the journey toward diabetes management and healthy living can actually help us feel better. When we live wellness-oriented lives, we live better. Finding praise and joy in our lives is simply easier when we have more energy, when we are less sick, and when we are really living.

*Loving God, I know that You have created me for life. Help me to live that life to the fullest and to enjoy this journey toward wellness. In Your holy name, Amen.*

# Day 14:
## Thanksgiving

## Morning Reflection

We have reached the end of week two in the journey toward diabetes management. Sometimes at this point, the journey can feel as if it is flying by, or it can feel like we are progressing at a snail's pace. The difficulties of the journey may weigh on us by now, or we may find the steps easier than we had expected. But whatever our experience to this point, today is a good day to stop, reflect, and give thanks.

### Faith Life
One of the most important aspects of our faith is thankfulness. Today make a list of the things for which you are thankful. At the end of the day, say a prayer, reading the list.

### Medical
Diabetes pills only work if you take them! If you have trouble remembering, try using a pill sorter box so that you will remember to take them every day.

### Movement
If you must stand in line when running errands, use the time to exercise your ankles and calves by doing some calf raises. Rise onto your toes and let yourself

back down. This will give you a little exercise and something to do while you stand in line.

## Work
When you get frustrated at work, take a moment to breathe. Take a deep breath, and say a short prayer of thanks. This can help you to take a step back and get some perspective before becoming overwhelmed.

## Emotional
Gratefulness is an attitude that we can practice. When we remember what we have been given, some of the things that cause us stress might not feel quite so big. Today when you start to feel stress, simply breathe and say the phrase, "I am grateful" before you move forward.

## Family and Friends
Are you thankful for your friends and family? Do they know it? Today take a moment and tell one (or more) of your friends and family that you are thankful for their presence in your life.

## Nutrition
So you know how much dressing you are getting, request salad dressing on the side of your salad when you eat out at a restaurant. Keep in mind that many dressings do come with sugar in them.

## Evening Wrap-up

*Shout for joy to the Lord, all the earth.*
*Worship the Lord with gladness; come before him*
*with joyful songs. . . . It is he who made us, and we*
*are his; we are his people, the sheep of his pasture.*
*Enter his gates with thanksgiving and his courts*
*with praise; give thanks to him and praise his name.*
*For the Lord is good and his love endures forever;*
*his faithfulness continues through all generations.*
PSALM 100

Thanksgiving is an important part of the wellness journey. When we take the time to give thanks, we take the time to evaluate where we are and recognize the good. As difficult as the road toward diabetes management and wellness can become, the psalmist reminds us that we belong to God and "his love endures forever." God is faithful and loves us, which is reason enough to be thankful.

*Lord God, You have given me so much for which to be*
*thankful. Help me today to take the time to be grateful.*
*In Your holy name, Amen.*

# Week 3

## Cindy's Story

When Cindy first came to the Church Health Center, she had been struggling with her weight for her entire life and struggling with diabetes for about ten years. She tried to lose weight and to get her diabetes under control. As she puts it, "I tried every diet known to man." But she never seemed able to stick to it. Her weight went up and down. She even tried starving herself, managing her portions to the point of obsession.

But even after losing weight, Cindy did not feel well. Discouraged, she went to her doctor, who put her on yet another medication to manage her diabetes. When Cindy expressed her frustration, her doctor recommended that she visit the Church Health Center.

She was skeptical at first: "I had convinced myself that I just couldn't lose weight and that I would always be sick."

But as she got into a regular exercise routine and attended some classes on diabetes management, Cindy began to feel better. She gradually learned the balance that worked for her. The weight started coming off, and more importantly, she started feeling better. Eventually she was weaned off several of her medications as her health improved.

Today she loves attending cooking classes, and she still exercises multiple times a week. She is managing her diabetes primarily with diet and exercise, and she feels great!

# Day 15:
# Balance

## Morning Reflection

Managing diabetes, like general wellness, is about balance. We have to find the right balance to maintain our blood glucose levels. We eat a balanced diet. We balance exercise with calorie intake. We even find it important to achieve a work-life balance, whatever that looks like. But with all the changes happening in our lives right now, it is sometimes easier to feel off balance than to feel like things are falling into place. So today we will focus on ways to stay balanced.

Faith Life

Go for a walking meditation today. Walk for about ten minutes around your house, around your block, or even around your workplace. As you walk, make an effort to notice the wonderful way that your body is put together and the balance that helps you walk.

Medical

Remember that medication is not magic. A lifestyle of diabetes management includes striking a balance between medications and lifestyle changes. At your next doctor's appointment, ask your doctor what changes you should be making in your life to be healthier.

## Movement
There is no movement without balance. Today spend two minutes balancing on one foot at a time. Balance as long as you can on one foot and then switch to the other, alternating for a total of ten minutes. By balancing you will build strength in your calves and ankles, as well as in your abdomen and back.

## Work
Many of us talk about finding the right "balance" between work and personal life. Today take five minutes and write about what the right balance looks like to you, whether or not you have currently achieved it.

## Emotional
Balancing busyness with downtime is very important to maintaining emotional wellness. Today take ten minutes to sit and relax. Take some deep breaths in and out. Close your eyes. Relax.

## Family and Friends
All of us can lose our balance from time to time. It is at those times when it is most important to reach out for support. Today go for a brisk walk with a friend or family member who might help support you on your journey.

## Nutrition

Good nutrition is mostly about balance and moderation. In particular, good nutrition includes appropriate portion sizes. Today keep a log of the things that you eat, and include the portion size. Remember that one portion of meat is about the size of a deck of cards.

## Evening Wrap-up

*"For I will pour water on the thirsty land,*
*and streams on the dry ground; I will pour out*
*my Spirit on your offspring, and my blessing on*
*your descendants. They will spring up like grass*
*in a meadow, like poplar trees by flowing streams.*
*Some will say, 'I belong to the LORD';*
*others will call themselves by the name of Jacob;*
*still others will write on their hand, 'The LORD's,'*
*and will take the name Israel."*
ISAIAH 44:3–5

Trying to change our routines and our habits means that our balance may be thrown off. Even if we are making positive changes, they are still *changes* and can impact our balance. But in this passage from Isaiah, we are assured that God cares for us, for we belong to the Lord. Even in the midst of change, God can help us find our right balance.

*Life-giving Lord, I know that I belong to You. I pray today that You would help me find my balance on this journey. In Your holy name, Amen.*

# Day 16:
## Grace

## Morning Reflection

Our culture often promotes the concept of "all or nothing," where if we are not giving 110 percent, then we have automatically failed. But managing diabetes simply does not work that way. During our first week, we looked at how we deal with setbacks, and one of the first steps is to acknowledge that setbacks do happen. On this journey, we will have good days and bad. But if we can manage to give ourselves some grace on the bad days, then we will make more progress than if we simply label bad days as "failures."

### Faith Life
Today read Matthew 19:26. Take five minutes and write about impossibility. Do any of your goals from week one feel impossible? How might God give you the grace to face even seemingly impossible tasks?

### Medical
Today begin keeping a list of questions that you can ask your doctor the next time you go in for a checkup. Put the list in an easy-to-find place, such as in your wallet or on your refrigerator.

## Movement
Today walk in place for five minutes and then try stretching for ten minutes. Try to touch your toes, reach your arms across your chest, stretch your back. If your muscles are cold, do not stretch too far!

## Work
Is your office break room always full of treats? Birthday cake, doughnuts, bagels? Offer a balance to some of these unhealthy snacks by bringing healthy snacks to share, such as a fruit and vegetable plate.

## Emotional
Learning to manage stress is very important to managing hypertension. Today take a slow walk, focusing on your breathing and letting go of the things that leave you overwhelmed.

## Family and Friends
Do you and your family have dinner together? Today plan a family dinner made up of mostly vegetables. Include a lean protein and a small serving of whole grains (such as brown rice, barley, or whole-wheat pasta).

## Nutrition
Do not skip meals! Skipping a meal can knock your blood sugar levels out of control and can make it difficult to get your glucose back to a normal level. If you know you are going to be on the road during your normal mealtime, pack a snack with carbohydrates and protein.

# Evening Wrap-up

*And God raised us up with Christ and seated us
with him in the heavenly realms in Christ Jesus,
in order that in the coming ages he might show
the incomparable riches of his grace, expressed in
his kindness to us in Christ Jesus. For it is by grace
you have been saved, through faith—and this is
not from yourselves, it is the gift of God.*
EPHESIANS 2:6–8

In his letter to the Ephesians, Paul reminds us of
the power of God's grace. We have been saved by
God's grace, though it is not earned. So if God offers
us such abundant grace, why can we not manage to
give ourselves some grace? The journey to wellness
and diabetes management is not about perfection.
It is instead about being as healthy as we can be for
the long haul.

*Gracious God, You offer me grace even when I do not
deserve it. Help me to give myself grace even on
the bad days as I continue on this journey.
In Your holy name, Amen.*

# Day 17:
## Senses

## Morning Reflection

Diabetes management and wellness are about much more than simply losing weight or switching to a new medication. The journey may certainly include some of these things, but wellness is a much larger picture than that. After all, we are created whole. We are given eyes to see and ears to hear. The world is full of beautiful things to see, taste, and touch. The journey to wellness is about embracing all of those senses.

Faith Life
Remember that God shows up in every aspect of our lives, including our food. Today before each meal, say a prayer. Thank God for the flavors and the colors in your food.

Medical
Remember that your current medical state is closely related to your family history. Today write out a brief medical history of your family. Pay special attention to diabetes. Keep your medical history on your refrigerator with your list of medications.

Movement
Go for a walk today and as you walk, observe all the colors, smells, and even tastes. Pay attention to the

air on your skin and the movement of your body. Say a prayer of thanks for all of those sensations as you move.

## Work
If you become bored at work today, try not to resort to eating. Instead take a moment and make a list of fifteen things that you can see, smell, feel, hear, or taste. Then say a small prayer of thanks.

## Emotional
When our emotions flare up and we become overwhelmed by stress, our blood sugar can go up. In managing diabetes, we must try to limit that surge of glucose. Today practice deep breathing to manage your blood glucose levels during times of stress.

## Family and Friends
Healthy relationships can bring balance to your life in many ways, but especially by offering fellowship and fun. Today call a friend or a family member and have some fun by dancing to some music or shopping at a farmer's market for some local fresh produce.

## Nutrition
Beware! Sugar is added to many things, such as soup, that we would not imagine. Today try adding flavor to your food by adding herbs and spices, such as basil, parsley, or rosemary. Add some flavor to a sandwich by adding watercress or cabbage instead of lettuce.

# Evening Wrap-up

*Jesus replied, "Go back and report to John what you hear and see: The blind receive sight, the lame walk, those who have leprosy are cleansed, the deaf hear, the dead are raised, and the good news is proclaimed to the poor. Blessed is anyone who does not stumble on account of me."*
MATTHEW 11:4–6

God created us with senses, and more than that, when God became human in the person of Jesus Christ, He restored our senses. Jesus restored sight to the blind and hearing to the deaf. We can know from this that those senses matter to God. They are an important part of who we are in God's creation. So on our journey to managing diabetes, we can find enjoyment, meaning, and balance in all of our senses.

*Loving God, You have given me the gift of senses. Help me today to enjoy the gift You have given me and to find my own balance in Your creation. In Your holy name, Amen.*

# Day 18:
## Out of the Comfort Zone

### Morning Reflection

The journey to diabetes management and wellness will undoubtedly take us outside of our comfort zone. That may mean cooking at home instead of stopping at the drive-through or ordering something completely different on a menu. But as we step outside that comfort zone, we occasionally need to be reminded that it is not necessarily unsafe, even if it is uncomfortable. Wherever we walk on this journey to wellness, God goes with us.

### Faith Life

Read Exodus 3, where God appears to Moses in the burning bush. When you have finished, spend five minutes writing about being called out of your comfort zone. Do you feel God's assurance, "I will be with you"?

### Medical

Make it a point to discuss "disaster plans" with your doctor. Make a list of things that you would need in the case of an emergency (insulin pens, medications, glucometer, glucose tablets).

## Movement

A healthy exercise regimen consists of building our aerobic strength, muscular strength, endurance, and flexibility. Today do three sets of ten wall push-ups to start building your upper-body strength.

## Work

When you begin to feel tired or bored at work, pay attention to your posture. Good posture helps you breathe, increases strength in your back and abdomen, and can give you a boost of energy when you need it.

## Emotional

Leaving your comfort zone can cause a great deal of anxiety or even panic. Today if you begin to feel anxious about leaving your comfort zone, slow down, take several deep breaths, and tell yourself out loud that you are safe.

## Family and Friends

Today go for a walk with your friends or family members. Set a goal for the walk that is slightly farther than you have walked before. Leaving your comfort zone can be less intimidating with friends and family around you.

## Nutrition

Eating a wellness-oriented diet means leaving behind food habits that may be comfortable and even comforting. Today try a new food, but don't forget to read the label!

# Evening Wrap-up

*But Moses said to God, "Who am I that I should go
to Pharaoh and bring the Israelites out of Egypt?"
And God said, "I will be with you. And this will
be the sign to you that it is I who have sent you:
When you have brought the people out of Egypt,
you will worship God on this mountain."*
EXODUS 3:11–12

God sometimes calls us out of our comfort zones and
routines. Moses was quite comfortable in Midian, but
God called him back to Egypt. Though we all know
the ending to that story now, at the time, Moses was
intimidated by the task put in front of him. But God
assured him, "I will be with you." Likewise, as we are
called to step outside of our comfort zones, God will
be with us.

*Lord God, give me courage and encouragement to make
the changes that I need to make in my life,
even as I leave my comfort zone.
In Your holy name, Amen.*

# Day 19:
## Purpose

## Morning Reflection

In our first week, we talked about foundations: the first building blocks to our journey. At this point, we are nearly halfway through the six-week journey, and it is a good time to revisit those foundations. Another way that we can talk about foundations is to return to an idea of purpose. Each of us has a different purpose for the journey, and at this point, halfway through, it is important for us to revisit that purpose.

### Faith Life
What were your goals for your faith life in week one? Today reread your goals, and then spend five minutes writing about your progress. Have any of your goals changed? Have you made progress where you hadn't expected it?

### Medical
When you pack a disaster kit, be sure to pack urine ketone testing strips as well as an insulated bag for insulin or other refrigerated medications in case of a power loss.

## Movement

In week one, you went for a walk. Go for a walk today. Do not exhaust yourself, but push yourself to walk as far as you can. Write in your journal about the progress that you have made.

## Work

Today take a copy of your list of prescriptions, vitamins, over-the-counter medications, and family history to keep at work. Keep the list in an accessible place.

## Emotional

Connecting with our purpose can help us gain stability and perspective as we go through periods of change. Today spend ten minutes writing in your journal about your purpose on this wellness journey.

## Family and Friends

Family and friends can be strong reminders of the purpose that we set for ourselves. Today have a healthy meal with your family or some friends and enjoy the social anchor that you have in your support system.

## Nutrition

What has changed in your diet since you started on this journey? Take a moment and write out your grocery list from this week. Compare it with the grocery list you made during week one. What has changed? What has remained the same?

## Evening Wrap-up

*Run in such a way as to get the prize.*
*Everyone who competes in the games goes*
*into strict training. They do it to get a crown*
*that will not last, but we do it to get a crown*
*that will last forever. Therefore I do not*
*run like someone running aimlessly;*
*I do not fight like a boxer beating the air.*
1 CORINTHIANS 9:24–26

Running a race without a goal or motivation makes little sense. In a similar fashion, walking the journey to diabetes management without an understanding of why we are doing it makes it more likely that, at the end of the day, we will not stick with our new lifestyle. In his letter to the Corinthians, Paul reminds us to run the race for the crown that will last. When we anchor our journey in the larger purpose, we are more likely to follow through to the end.

*Loving God, give me the vision today to seek the crown that will last. In Your holy name, Amen.*

# Day 20:
# Change

## Morning Reflection

As we have seen, we all have patterns and habits that can be quite difficult to change. But change is a part of life. All of us change as we grow—we age, change jobs, and move to different cities. But regardless of the inevitability of change, it is still stressful at times. Even change that is desired can make us feel off balance. On this journey, we are actively working to alter our lives, and while we make those changes, it is entirely possible that we will lose our center for a while.

### Faith Life
Do you have a "go-to" Bible verse that you return to when you need encouragement? Today spend ten minutes reflecting on that one verse that anchors you. Remember that you have anchors even in the midst of change.

### Medical
If possible, find a place at work where you can keep medication that you need during the day, instead of taking your medication with you to work each day. Make sure it is well labeled!

## Movement
Today if you are running errands, park your car in the parking space farthest away from the entrance to the store. Add steps to your day by forcing yourself to walk farther.

## Work
When work becomes stressful, it is easy to turn to food without even recognizing what you are doing. Today if you start to feel overwhelmed at work, don't head for the vending machines, head for the door! Take a short break outside, breathe in some fresh air, and let your body relax before getting back to work.

## Emotional
Many of us in the past have dealt with the discomfort of change by eating. Today make a list of things that you can do to give yourself comfort that will help on your journey. Go for a walk, for example, or read a book.

## Family and Friends
When was the last time you let your friends know how important they are to you? Today let them know. Write your friends a note, e-mail, text message, or just call them on the phone.

## Nutrition
Salads are definitely healthy, but be careful of the dressing and cheese! Many dressings have a great deal of sugar, fat, and extra calories. Use low-fat

cheese, and substitute cream-based or mayonnaise-based dressings (like ranch or thousand island) for a vinaigrette or even just some vinegar and oil with a little pepper and oregano.

## Evening Wrap-up

*"Do not fear, for I have redeemed you;*
*I have summoned you by name; you are mine.*
*When you pass through the waters,*
*I will be with you; and when you pass through*
*the rivers, they will not sweep over you.*
*When you walk through the fire, you will not be*
*burned; the flames will not set you ablaze."*
ISAIAH 43:1–2

When we encounter change in our lives—whether we asked for it or not—we can feel like we have been thrown into chaos. We can no longer rely on our old habits and structures to hold us up. In this passage from Isaiah, we are assured that in the midst of chaos, we belong to God. On this journey to diabetes management and wellness, we can remember that we still belong to God, even when we feel we are in the midst of chaos.

*God in our midst, I know that I belong—body and spirit—to You. Help me to cling to You even in times of change and fear. In Your holy name, Amen.*

# Day 21:
# Halfway

## Morning Reflection

Congratulations! Today marks the halfway point on our six-week journey. We know, of course, that the journey toward wellness and diabetes management is a lifelong journey. But today we can celebrate a milestone on our current leg of the journey together. While the halfway point is certainly something to celebrate, it can also be daunting at times. We can both look back on the progress that we have made and look ahead and see the road still ahead of us.

### Faith Life
Endurance comes with peace, and peace comes with quiet. Today practice sitting quietly. Take five minutes, sit quietly, and breathe. Reflect on the journey to this point and how God has been present with you.

### Medical
What are your long-term health goals? Keep in mind that quick fixes in medicine are generally not long-term solutions. The next time you have a doctor's appointment, talk to your care provider about your long-term health goals.

### Movement
Today do some jumping jacks. Try a set of fifteen, take a one-minute break, and then do it again. Try

that three times throughout the day. Remember that in order to build endurance, we must occasionally push limits.

## Work
When you take your break at work, do you crave a specific food? This may be habitual eating. Today if you feel hungry at work, drink some water, or snack on some chopped fresh vegetables instead of heading for the vending machines.

## Emotional
Marathon runners will tell you that endurance is at least as emotional as it is physical. Today spend five minutes breathing and repeat to yourself that you can continue on this journey. Try not to tell yourself that this is something that you cannot do.

## Family and Friends
Friends are so important to give us encouragement while we are on the journey. Today schedule a dinner with some of your friends who will give you encouragement.

## Nutrition
Managing diabetes does not mean giving up desserts completely! Instead of a dessert rich in sugar and fat, try grilling some fruit kabobs and eating them with low-fat yogurt or low-fat ricotta cheese. Grilling the fruit will bring some of the natural sugars to the surface and will add a little natural sweetness.

## Evening Wrap-up

*Then we will no longer be infants, tossed back and forth by the waves. . . . Instead, speaking the truth in love, we will grow to become in every respect the mature body of him who is the head, that is, Christ. From him the whole body, joined and held together by every supporting ligament, grows and builds itself up in love, as each part does its work.*
EPHESIANS 4:14–16

As we continue on this journey to diabetes management and wellness, we are growing and maturing. Our bodies are transforming, and our relationships to our bodies are changing. Halfway through this six-week journey, we may be daunted by the path still ahead of us, but we can look back and celebrate our accomplishments so far. Furthermore, we can rest assured in the knowledge that God is with us.

*Loving God, thank You for walking with me all this way. Continue to be with me as I press on toward the goal. In Your holy name, Amen.*

# Week 4

## Tony's Story

When Tony began his journey with the Church Health Center, he was feeling pretty helpless. He thought that there was very little that he or anyone else could do to get his health under control. But at the advice of his doctor, he decided to take a Healthy Bodies class, and he started getting regular exercise three times a week.

"I had never really taken the time to consider that my health problems were in any way connected to my faith life. I had kept the two completely separate."

As he exercised and learned more about nutrition and diabetes management, Tony lost some weight (about ten pounds) and was feeling healthier. His blood pressure went down as well.

But what really made the difference, according to Tony, was the way he began to understand his body in relationship to God. "I came to realize that my body belongs to God, and it's mine to take care of for the time being." That understanding gave Tony motivation to get—and keep—his diabetes under control.

Today Tony is still taking classes and exercising at least three times a week. His diabetes is under control, and he has more energy to spend with his grandkids.

# Day 22:
## God's Creation

## Morning Reflection

When we set out on the journey to diabetes management and wellness, it is often with the attitude that we are making choices about our individual health. While this is true, it is also not the entire picture. We have been created by God. As such, we are not merely individuals, but we are a part of God's creation—that very creation of which we are stewards. When we care for our bodies, we care for God's creation.

### Faith Life
Psalm 34:8 reads, "Taste and see that the Lord is good; blessed is the one who takes refuge in him." Take five minutes and write about finding God in many aspects of creation, even your food.

### Medical
We all get sick, and that is particularly complicated for diabetics. Do you have a plan for sick days? This week we will focus on making that plan. Today locate a place where you can write out your sick-day plan.

## Movement
Go for a walk outside today. As you walk, focus on your breathing. Try to inhale as you take three steps and exhale as you take three steps.

## Work
Are you able to see outside from your place of work? Today bring some inspiring pictures to work to give you a break from the indoors when you need it.

## Emotional
Today practice managing your stress with slow, deep breathing. Relax your shoulders, lift your chin, close your eyes, and take a deep breath using your abdominal muscles. Hold your breath in for three seconds, then slowly let your breath out.

## Family and Friends
Today go to a park with your family and friends. Enjoy being outside in God's creation with them. Instead of focusing on food, focus on the fun and beauty of creation.

## Nutrition
When you shop, look for bread that contains "whole wheat flour" or "whole grain" in the ingredients. If the label just says "wheat," it's not a whole grain product.

## Evening Wrap-up

*Then the L*ORD *spoke to Job out of the storm.*
*He said. . . "Where were you when I laid the*
*earth's foundation? Tell me, if you understand.*
*Who marked off its dimensions? Surely you know!*
*Who stretched a measuring line across it? On what*
*were its footings set, or who laid its cornerstone—*
*while the morning stars sang together*
*and all the angels shouted for joy?"*
JOB 38:1, 4–7

Job was considered the most righteous of God's
servants, and yet, Job needed to be reminded of
his own place in creation. That is, Job was a part
of creation, not the whole of it. God spoke to Job,
reminding him of just how comprehensive creation
is, and how intricately God has created the world.
Likewise on our journey to diabetes management,
we would do well to remember and recognize the
intricacy of God's creation and the place of our own
bodies within that creation.

*Loving God, I know that You laid the earth's foundation.*
*Help me today to see Your creation in myself.*
*In Your holy name, Amen.*

# Day 23:
## Sun

## Morning Reflection

As children, many of us loved spending time in the sun—playing outdoors or swimming in a pool. But as adults, the sun often becomes an object of nuisance and even fear. But how often do we stop and appreciate the wonders of the sun? The sun allows us the wonderful food that we eat. The sun provides warmth and light. Today we will focus on ways that we can incorporate the sun into our journey toward diabetes management.

### Faith Life
Today try to find an unusual place to pray. Pray while waiting in line, while you're stuck in traffic, or while you're on hold with someone on the phone. Take just a moment and offer a short prayer to God, perhaps, "God, thank You for the gift of light."

### Medical
Illness puts you in a state of stress, which can raise your blood sugar. If you are sick, make sure that you drink fluids, even if you cannot eat. Each hour, try to drink eight ounces of sugar-free, caffeine-free drinks, such as water or tea (without milk).

## Movement
Spend some time outside today walking or even going for a light jog. Even if it is cold outside, put on some layers and get outdoors. Remember to wear sunscreen!

## Work
Enjoying the sun can be particularly difficult at our jobs, but our work is not just at our job. Today do some work outside. Wash your car, mow your lawn, or work in your garden. You'll get some sun and some exercise!

## Emotional
The sun can provide a much-needed emotional lift, as well as vitamin D. Today find ten minutes to sit outside in the sun and practice deep breathing. Feel the sun's warmth, and try to let your body relax as you sit.

## Family and Friends
Go for a walk outside with a friend or family member. Try to enjoy the outdoors and the company of someone who cares for you.

## Nutrition
Today add a serving of nonstarchy vegetables to each of your meals. Add spinach to your breakfast eggs, a serving of raw carrots to your lunch, and some sautéed cucumbers to your dinner.

## Evening Wrap-up

*And God said, "Let there be light," and there
was light. God saw that the light was good,
and he separated the light from the darkness.
God called the light "day," and the darkness
he called "night." And there was evening,
and there was morning—the first day.*
GENESIS 1:3–5

The sun often gets a bad rap in our culture today.
Many of us do not have time to get outside and
enjoy the warmth of the sun on our skin, and when
we do have the time, we view the sun as an enemy.
But in reality, while we need to be cautious about
our sun exposure, we will be healthier if we can find
safe ways to enjoy the sun. Furthermore, by enjoying the sun responsibly, we can truly embrace and
enjoy God's creation.

*Glorious God, You made the sun as a beautiful part of Your
creation. Today help me to enjoy the light that You have
given me, as well as the fruits and vegetables that are
possible because of Your light. In Your holy name, Amen.*

# Day 24:
## Air

## Morning Reflection

In the morning when we wake up, many of us yawn and stretch before we are even fully conscious. We take a deep breath, filling our lungs with fresh morning air before we set foot on the floor of our bedroom. The air that we breathe is so important, and yet most of the time we take it for granted. Today we will focus on how we can have a relationship with air that will help us on the journey to diabetes management.

### Faith Life
There are dozens of verses in the Bible about how God uses the wind. Today read John 3:8, and when you encounter the wind today take it as a reminder of God's Spirit moving in the world.

### Medical
When you are sick, monitoring your blood sugar is particularly important. If you are not feeling well, check your glucose every two to four hours, particularly if you are vomiting or have diarrhea.

## Movement
Today try to walk someplace where you would normally drive. Get some great exercise by walking, and keep just a little of those pollutants from getting into the air.

## Work
If you feel anxiety at work, try to do some deep breathing. Take just a minute and focus on controlling your breathing. It will help to lessen your anxiety and will give you a boost of energy and focus.

## Emotional
Air is a very important part of stress relief. Today spend five minutes sitting with your back straight, breathing. Breathe in through your nose and out through your mouth. If you start to feel lightheaded, try to relax your chest and stomach muscles.

## Family and Friends
Prepare a meal today with your family or friends and enjoy all the aromas that you produce in the kitchen. The smells of food all come from the gift of air.

## Nutrition
When you look at your plate at mealtime, most of the plate should be occupied by nonstarchy vegetables, such as leafy greens, broccoli, or mushrooms. Today take a look at your plate. How much of your plate is taken up with vegetables?

## Evening Wrap-up

*And God said, "Let there be a vault between the waters to separate water from water." So God made the vault and separated the water under the vault from the water above it. And it was so. God called the vault "sky." And there was evening, and there was morning—the second day.*
GENESIS 1:6–8

When we think of diabetes management, we do not immediately think of breathing. But the journey to diabetes management is a journey toward overall wellness, and the air that we breathe is absolutely an important piece of wellness. While our journey to wellness is dependent on the air that we breathe, we often take it for granted. When do we notice the air—when it smells bad or when the wind is blowing. But God has given us the air as a part of creation—to breathe, to enjoy, and to cherish.

*Loving God, You have given me the air to breathe.
Help me to slow down and appreciate
the wonders of Your creation.
In Your holy name, Amen.*

# Day 25:
## Water

---

## Morning Reflection

Most of us know, on some level, just how important water is to our lives. Water covers about 70 percent of the earth's surface and makes up more than half of our own bodies. Water gives us options for fun and recreation in the form of swimming, boating, and playing in the sprinklers, to name a few. Water also nourishes plants and vegetables, giving us not only food, but also lush trees and flowers. So water is a wonderful gift, and yet, most wellness experts agree that we do not drink enough of it. Today we will focus on God's gift of water.

### Faith Life
The next time it rains, try to think of the rain as a blessing. Today write a prayer thanking God for the blessing of water.

### Medical
When you are sick, every third hour or so, try to drink eight ounces of caffeine-free liquid. If you are sick to your stomach, take the liquid in small sips to help with your nausea.

### Movement
Swimming is excellent exercise. It is gentle on your joints and works just about every muscle group in

your body. Today if you have access to a pool, go for a swim—even spending ten minutes in the water will give you some great exercise.

## Work

Instead of drinking soda today, try drinking water. The sugar and caffeine in soda can actually leave you dehydrated and feeling lethargic. Water will replenish your bodily fluids and will actually leave you with more and lasting energy, instead of just a sugar rush.

## Emotional

Most of us shower in the morning. Today to relax, take a five-minute shower at the end of the day. The noise from the shower will help to drown out the noise of the day, and the heat from the water will help to relax your muscles.

## Family and Friends

Serving water with meals is a great way to meet your daily water goals (at least eight eight-ounce glasses). Today when you have dinner with your family, put a pitcher of water on the table with the rest of the meal.

## Nutrition

If you are getting tired of drinking water, try adding a lemon or a lime to your glass, or use a sugar-free additive to make your water taste sweeter. Even the occasional sugar-free soda can add some variety—but if you add a soda, make sure that it does not "replace" a glass of water!

# Evening Wrap-up

*And God said, "Let the water under the sky*
*be gathered to one place, and let dry ground*
*appear." And it was so. God called the dry ground*
*"land," and the gathered waters he called "seas."*
*And God saw that it was good.*
GENESIS 1:9–10

Water is everywhere—not only in God's creation,
but also throughout the Bible. We hear about the
destructive power of water in the story of the Great
Flood, but also the regenerative power of water in
baptism. Water is powerful and life giving, and it is
a sign of God's love and care for creation. So as we
move forward on our journey to wellness and diabetes management, we can appreciate the beauty
and the power of God's creation through water.

*Loving God, You created water, and You made water a part*
*of me. I pray today that You would help me to appreciate*
*the beauty and power of water on the earth and in me.*
*In Your holy name, Amen.*

# Day 26:
## Land

## Morning Reflection

Take a moment, close your eyes, and let your mind picture "God's creation." Most likely, you have in mind some piece of land: majestic mountains, lush forests, colorful flowers, even a desert. The land has been created by God to offer a huge variety of plants and animals that we can enjoy. And yet, most of us have very little connection to where our food actually comes from. Today we will explore the beautiful and bountiful land that God has created.

### Faith Life
When you sit down to eat a meal, do you see God's creation? Today when you sit down to meals, try to imagine where each piece of your meal came from, and give thanks for each item.

### Medical
If your blood sugar is running low when you are sick, try drinking a cup of sports drink or half a cup of fruit juice. Avoid caffeine.

### Movement
Gardening can provide great exercise. If you do not have the space to enjoy a full garden, try planting

some tomatoes or herbs in pots. This way you can both enjoy gardening and fresh herbs or vegetables.

## Work
Do your coworkers know about your journey to wellness? Today tell at least one of your coworkers about your goals. Often workplaces can come together to strive toward wellness as a community.

## Emotional
Being a member of a community is a very important part of emotional wellness as well as physical wellness. Today instead of spending time writing in your journal, spend at least ten minutes sitting with someone who is a member of your support system, and talk to him or her.

## Family and Friends
A farmer's market can be a great way to find affordable local produce, and a great place to spend some time with friends and family. (Often there is live music or other entertainment.) Today take a few minutes and see if your town has a farmer's market.

## Nutrition
The fresher your food, the healthier it is. If you cannot find a vegetable in the fresh produce section, try the frozen food section. "Flash-frozen" fruits and vegetables are just as nutritious as fresh vegetables and can be used in the same recipes.

## Evening Wrap-up

*Then God said, "Let the land produce vegetation:*
*seed-bearing plants and trees on the land*
*that bear fruit with seed in it, according to their*
*various kinds." And it was so. The land produced*
*vegetation: plants bearing seed according*
*to their kinds and trees bearing fruit with*
*seed in it according to their kinds.*
*And God saw that it was good.*
GENESIS 1:11–13

We are learning different habits. In some cases, this means learning how to relate differently to God's creation. On this journey, we can learn how to appreciate the wonderful gifts that God has given us. We are also learning how to incorporate the wonders of God's creation into our refrigerators and onto our dinner tables. When we work to appreciate the wonder of God's creation, we work toward lasting wellness.

*God of Creation, on my journey to diabetes management,*
*help me to more fully incorporate the bounty of*
*Your creation into my life and onto my table.*
*In Your holy name, Amen.*

# Day 27:
## Bodies

## Morning Reflection

This week we have turned our focus to our relationships with God's creation. We have considered many of the external factors of God's creation. Today we arrive at yet another crucial aspect of God's creation: our own bodies. Yesterday we imagined God's creation, but chances are, very few of us actually pictured our own bodies as a part of God's creation. Yet our bodies are created and cared for by God, just as the sun and the land are.

### Faith Life
Today when you pray, pray a movement prayer. Stretch out your arms. Touch your toes. Stretch your neck. Feel the brilliance in God's creation and the way that your body is put together.

### Medical
When you are not feeling well, take your temperature. A fever can dehydrate you and put your body under more stress than normal.

### Movement
Today go for a brisk walk, and when you are finished, spend at least five minutes stretching. Try to feel and stretch as many muscles in your body as possible.

## Work
Work often requires repeating the same motion over and over again. When you take a break, spend five minutes doing something completely different than what you usually do. For example, if you sit at a computer typing most of the day, stand up and do jumping jacks.

## Emotional
Our emotions are more tied up with our bodies than we usually realize. Today spend five minutes smiling, even if you do not feel like smiling. Chances are you will feel a little better at the end of those five minutes.

## Family and Friends
Many of our self-esteem issues come from directing hatred toward our own bodies. Today ask a friend or family member to tell you what they like about your body.

## Nutrition
When you sit down to a meal, one quarter of your plate should be starchy foods, such as whole-grain rice, beans, or potatoes. Today take a look at your plate. How much of your plate is occupied by starchy foods?

# Evening Wrap-up

*Jesus said to them, "Come and have breakfast."*
*None of the disciples dared ask him,*
*"Who are you?" They knew it was the Lord.*
*Jesus came, took the bread and gave it to them,*
*and did the same with the fish.*
*This was now the third time Jesus appeared to his*
*disciples after he was raised from the dead.*
JOHN 21:12–14

Many of us do not have a particularly loving relationship with our bodies. But God has created our bodies and cares enough about them that when God became human in Jesus, He came in a body—twice! In this passage from John, Jesus appears to the disciples after the resurrection and asks them to have breakfast with Him. This meal on the beach is a story told to let us know that the resurrected Jesus was not a ghost but was flesh and bone!

*Loving God, You know what it is to have a body.*
*Help me to love and appreciate my body as a part of*
*Your creation on this journey. In Your holy name, Amen.*

# Day 28:
## Spirits

## Morning Reflection

Congratulations! We have made it to the end of the fourth week. At this point on the journey to diabetes management, we are making gradual but significant changes to our lifestyle. But as we make physical and external changes to our exercise routines and nutrition, we may also be noticing a transformation in our spirits. Our spirits, too, are a part of God's creation. When we read about God's creation of Adam, Adam did not become a man until God breathed the breath of life into him. As a part of God's creation, we are called to care for our spirits as well as our bodies.

Faith Life
What do you think a healthy spirit is? Today take ten minutes to pray and then write a few sentences about what having a healthy spirit means to you.

Medical
Today set aside a place in your pantry (or in a closet) for sick-day supplies. Include both sugar-free and sweetened gelatin, a box of instant broth, a bottle of apple juice, urine ketone testing strips, and a thermometer.

## Movement

Helping out a neighbor with yard work or even moving is a wonderful act of kindness and generosity, and it can get your heart rate up and burn calories, to boot! Today try to help a friend, family member, or neighbor with a project.

## Work

If you find yourself standing in one place for a period of time (making copies, talking on the phone, waiting for lunch to heat up), spend that time doing squats.

## Emotional

We often expect perfection of ourselves. The trouble with such expectations is that we are simply not perfect, and we can become demoralized. Today write for ten minutes about a time that you expected perfection from yourself.

## Family and Friends

Today recruit some family members and friends to help you with a project that you have been putting off—rearranging furniture, painting a room, mowing the lawn. Getting things accomplished is a great way to bond and lift spirits generally.

## Nutrition

Avoid frying vegetables or cooking them in cream sauces. Try using healthier preparation, such as grilling, baking, or steaming. This will help to maintain maximum flavor without adding extra fat, salt, and cholesterol.

## Evening Wrap-up

*For those who are led by the Spirit of God are the children of God. The Spirit you received does not make you slaves, so that you live in fear again; rather, the Spirit you received brought about your adoption to sonship. And by him we cry, "Abba, Father." The Spirit himself testifies with our spirit that we are God's children.*
ROMANS 8:14–16

On this journey to diabetes management, we are working to transform ourselves physically and spiritually. We are becoming more physically active, changing our nutritional habits, and hopefully, we are beginning to feel better. When we feel physically better, our spirits are lighter. Paul reminds us of the importance of our relationship to our spirit, and God's relationship to our spirit. We are God's children through our spirits, and God cares for us.

*Abba God, I know You have created me—body and spirit. Help me today and on this entire journey toward diabetes management to feel better and lighter in spirit. In Your holy name, Amen.*

# Week 5

## Anna's Story

Anna had been a diabetic for most of her adult life. She was consistently about seventy-five pounds overweight, and despite her many efforts, never managed to stick with any particular diet plan or lifestyle change. "I was eating unhealthy food most of the time. Every time I tried to get healthy, I would do well for about a week, and then something would happen. Sometimes, I just got bored."

But when Anna's doctor put her on yet another medication to manage her glucose levels, she decided to get serious. "I went to the Church Health Center, and I realized that I wasn't doing myself any favors by eating the way I was eating." Anna found, through classes and experimenting in her own kitchen, that living a wellness-oriented lifestyle and managing her diabetes did not have to be boring. She started exercising three times a week, and she kept a log to track her carbohydrate intake. She switched to eating whole grains and added many vegetables to her diet.

Over the course of two years, Anna lost fifty pounds and reduced her number of medications from four to one. She loves experimenting with new recipes and continues to exercise four or five times a week. "I thank God that I'm finally feeling good," she says.

# Day 29:
# Variety

## Morning Reflection

There is a common misconception that wellness is necessarily bland. We picture a leaf of lettuce on a plate with no dressing, endless hours on a treadmill, and of course, no salt, butter, or sugar. But in reality, wellness is about finding the rich variety already present in our lives. God has blessed us with a beautiful variety in the wonders of creation. So this week we will focus on the ways that variety can enhance our journey toward diabetes management.

### Faith Life

We have all had some variety and change in our faith life. Take ten minutes today and write about a time in your faith journey when you started heading in one direction but life or God pointed you down an unexpected path.

### Medical

Are you on medications? Have you been feeling better? Do not stop taking any medications until you have discussed it with your primary care provider. Stopping medication suddenly can lead to relapse, drug resistance, or unexpected side effects.

## Movement
Aim to exercise one to two hours after a meal, when your blood sugar is highest. If you cannot exercise then, be sure to check your glucose level. If it is under one hundred, eat a snack, such as half a sandwich with four ounces of juice.

## Work
During your lunch break at work, find some stairs and climb up and down them several times. This gives you a great aerobic workout without your even needing to go to the gym. (Hint: DO NOT skip your lunch to exercise!)

## Emotional
We are approaching the end of this six-week journey. Do you have different expectations now than you did when you started? Spend five minutes today writing about your current expectations for the journey.

## Family and Friends
Family and friends can be our constants when other things in life are unpredictable. Today make a healthy meal for your family or friends. Enjoy the food, but focus on the company and conversation.

## Nutrition
Meat can be a wonderful source of protein, but it can also be a source of fat and cholesterol. Today try to go the entire day without adding meat. Try some vegetarian recipes using beans, nuts, or soy for protein.

## Evening Wrap-up

*Praise the LORD from the earth, you great sea
creatures and all ocean depths, lightning and hail,
snow and clouds, stormy winds that do his
bidding, you mountains and all hills, fruit trees
and all cedars, wild animals and all cattle, small
creatures and flying birds, kings of the earth and
all nations, you princes and all rulers on earth,
young men and women, old men and children.*
PSALM 148:7–12

We have now arrived at week five, and at this point, we are beginning the descent from the summit of the mountain. But as we move forward, even as we look to the conclusion of this particular journey, we continue to be assured that God walks with us. We are reminded of God's presence with us every time we look around. The psalmist reminds us of the diversity of God's creation and the variety of our surroundings.

*God of creation, I know that You have made the world
and all its variety, and I pray that You would continue
to walk with me. In Your holy name, Amen.*

# Day 30:
# God in Our Midst

## Morning Reflection

The path to diabetes management includes many changes that can truly throw a loop into our sense of stability and consistency. That is not to say that it is all bad (or even bad at all). However, when faced with all of the changes that are part of this journey, finding a point to hold on to can help us feel steady. We have been saying throughout the weeks thus far that God walks this journey with us, and that is as true today as it was five weeks ago.

### Faith Life
Take ten minutes today to reflect on and write about the darkest moment in your faith life. Did God find you there? How?

### Medical
While it is sometimes important to lose weight in order to manage your diabetes, it is also possible to lose weight too quickly, resulting in malnutrition and loss of muscle and bone mass. Talk with your doctor or medical expert about setting healthy and reasonable weight-loss goals.

## Movement
This week try stepping up your aerobic exercise by doing ten jumping jacks before you go out for a walk and when you get back. This will help to get your heart rate up so you start out your walk with a higher heart rate.

## Work
Instead of going out to eat or getting lunch from a vending machine, bring in a lunch made from your leftovers from last night's dinner. It is almost guaranteed to be healthier, and it is much less expensive!

## Emotional
Have you had any setbacks recently? Today take five minutes to write about your setbacks, and then let them go. Move forward from here.

## Family and Friends
Soon these six weeks will be done, and it will be time to find your own rhythms and patterns. Today write down the names of a few friends or family members who might be willing to join you on the journey to wellness.

## Nutrition
Some fats are necessary for balanced nutrition. Healthy fats can be found in avocados, seeds and nuts, olive oil, and fish. Today prepare a meal using mostly healthy fats (no fried food or butter).

# Evening Wrap-up

*Love one another deeply. . . . For you have
been born again, not of perishable seed,
but of imperishable, through the living and
enduring word of God. . . . Therefore, rid yourselves of all malice and all deceit, hypocrisy, envy,
and slander of every kind. Like newborn babies,
crave pure spiritual milk, so that by it you may
grow up in your salvation, now that you have
tasted that the Lord is good.*
1 PETER 1:22–2:3

Psalm 34 tells us to "taste and see" the goodness
of God. Here, in this passage from 1 Peter, we are
told that we can taste that the Lord is good. God is
present in each of our senses, and we can find God
on our dinner tables. We can taste God's goodness
coming through each bite of a carefully prepared
meal. And so we are reminded each day of God's
presence with us on this journey.

*Loving God, I know that You are good,
and I pray today that You would give me the wisdom
to recognize Your presence with me on this journey.
In Your holy name, Amen.*

# Day 31:
## The Seasons

## Morning Reflection

The journey toward wellness and diabetes management is made up of seasons, just like a year is made up of seasons. Each season has its advantages and disadvantages, things we like and things we do not like. But we also know that in each season, we are presented with opportunities to encounter God in unique ways. Each season gives us a new opportunity to grow and learn and change on the journey.

### Faith Life
We can see God in all the seasons, wherever we are. But sometimes it is easier than other times. In which season can you see God most easily? Take five minutes and write a prayer for that season.

### Medical
Do you have any wounds or sores that are taking a long time to heal? Even if they do not hurt, sores that are not healing, especially on your feet, should be seen right away by your doctor.

### Movement
Different seasons allow for different kinds of exercise. During the summer, you can go swimming. In the autumn, you can play in the leaves. In winter,

you can shovel snow. Today try to engage in a season-specific activity.

## Work
Most workplaces have periods that are busy and periods that are slower. Whatever your work environment is like at this moment, find five minutes to breathe and stretch a little.

## Emotional
Do you expect your lifestyle changes to be all-or-nothing? Today take five minutes to write in your journal, reminding yourself that setbacks and individual "failures" are just seasons. If we persevere, they pass.

## Family and Friends
Are there seasons (such as the holiday season) when you spend more time with your family? Take a few minutes today and brainstorm some ways to make your family gatherings healthier, knowing what you know now about wellness.

## Nutrition
A wonderful way to add variety to your diet is to buy seasonal fruits and vegetables. They will be fresher than out-of-season produce, and they will also cost less.

## Evening Wrap-up

*"He changes times and seasons; he deposes kings and raises up others. He gives wisdom to the wise and knowledge to the discerning. He reveals deep and hidden things; he knows what lies in darkness, and light dwells with him. I thank and praise you, God of my ancestors: You have given me wisdom and power, you have made known to me what we asked of you, you have made known to us the dream of the king."*
DANIEL 2:21–23

We have seasons of new growth and seasons of harvest. But whatever the season that we are passing through, we can know that God is walking with us. After all, Daniel tells us that God changes times and seasons. God walks with us through each of our own seasons of coolness and warmth, birth and rebirth.

*Loving God, You change the times and seasons.
Your power inspires me on this journey.
I pray that You would continue to walk through my seasons on this journey with me. In Your holy name, Amen.*

# Day 32:
## Variety in Sound

## Morning Reflection

Each day we are surrounded by sound from the moment we wake up to the moment we fall asleep at night. It is only very, very rarely that any of us truly encounters silence, because God's creation is a noisy one! Though for the most part, we tend to ignore a majority of the sounds that we hear, we do hear a great variety of sounds throughout the day. And those sounds can be a wonderful part of our journey to diabetes management and wellness.

### Faith Life
What is your favorite sound in the world? Today write for five minutes about that sound. What does the sound remind you of? Where does God fit into that sound?

### Medical
When was the last time you went to the dentist? People with diabetes are more at risk for oral health problems such as gum disease. If it has been more than six months, call and make an appointment today.

## Movement
Make sure that you have well-fitting shoes for exercising. Many foot ulcers are caused by shoes that are too tight. If you are unsure of how a shoe should fit, ask your doctor or podiatrist.

## Work
If it is appropriate, put on some soft music while you work, using either small speakers or headphones. Listening to music can help to pass time and can also lift your mood or relax you.

## Emotional
Sound can help you identify and deal with your moods. Today take five minutes and write down ten sounds that you find comforting and calming. The next time you feel overwhelmed or stressed, imagine one of those sounds to calm down.

## Family and Friends
When you gather family and friends for a holiday or special occasion, think about playing games instead of focusing entirely on food. That way the gathering is more about being in each other's company than eating.

## Nutrition
Beware of frozen dinners. As quick as they may be, they are often loaded with sodium and sugar. Sometimes the diet versions are a little better, but there is no guarantee. Be sure to read the labels before consuming.

# Evening Wrap-up

*Shout for joy to the LORD, all the earth, burst into jubilant song with music; make music to the LORD with the harp, with the harp and the sound of singing, with trumpets and the blast of the ram's horn—shout for joy before the LORD, the King. Let the sea resound, and everything in it, the world, and all who live in it. Let the rivers clap their hands, let the mountains sing together for joy; let them sing before the LORD, for he comes to judge the earth."*
PSALM 98:4–9

Sounds can be reminders of God's grace and presence in our lives. Noises can also be ways that we can praise and worship God. The psalmist writes, "Make a joyful noise." Can there be a more joyful noise than a healthy person moving and enjoying the movement? What would happen if we considered the sound of our feet on the pavement on the same level as praise and worship songs? (We would probably walk a little more!) As we move forward, let us remember that God loves us and wants us to be healthy.

*Living God, thank You for the gift of sound.*
*Help me listen more carefully on this journey*
*to weight management. In Your holy name, Amen.*

# Day 33:
## Variety in Sight

## Morning Reflection

Each time we open our eyes, we encounter a multitude of sights. God has given us the gift of variety in sight. But God has also given us the gift of seeing differently. Have you ever had the experience of looking at a tree or a building—one that you have seen dozens of times—and suddenly feeling like you are seeing it for the first time? On this journey to diabetes management, our vision is changing. We are coming to see wellness differently.

### Faith Life
Do you have potluck dinners at your church? Next time try bringing a healthy dish instead of a typical dish. For example, bring fresh fruit salad instead of a pie.

### Medical
Today take a few minutes to critique your vision and if necessary, make an appointment to have your eyes checked or your prescription updated. Also keep in mind that diabetes can cause vision problems, and let your eye-care professional know about your diabetes.

## Movement

Go for a walk today. Walk for as long as you can manage and take in the sights of the world around you. Try to notice the difference in your walking now from when you started.

## Work

Coffee tends to be a staple of our workday, but too often we add heavy creams or lots of sugar to sweeten our coffee. Today instead of coffee, try an herbal tea. Rather than adding cream or sugar, let the flavors in the tea serve to sweeten the experience.

## Emotional

Do you have any visual cues that are connected to your emotional state? For example, what do you feel when you look out the window and see snow? Or the sight of a fire in the fireplace? Today take five minutes and write about some of the most emotionally powerful images in your life.

## Family and Friends

Today for fun get out some old pictures of you and your family. Let the pictures inspire storytelling and camaraderie around a healthy meal.

## Nutrition

Substitute, don't add. If you really want to have a cookie or a piece of cake, substitute that for another carbohydrate that you would have eaten that day. For example, replace your baked potato with a cookie for dessert.

## Evening Wrap-up

*How abundant are the good things that you have stored up for those who fear you, that you bestow in the sight of all, on those who take refuge in you. In the shelter of your presence you hide them from all human intrigues; you keep them safe in your dwelling from accusing tongues. Praise be to the LORD, for he showed me the wonders of his love.*
PSALM 31:19–21

We are working to change the way that we see ourselves. In particular, we are working to see ourselves the way God sees us. God loves us and cares for us. God has created us—body and spirit. On this journey, we are learning to see ourselves as God's creations. Our sight is being restored by the God who created us.

*Loving God, You have created me, and I know that You love and care for me. I pray that You would give me the vision to see You in myself. In Your holy name, Amen.*

# Day 34:
## The Fruits of Wellness

## Morning Reflection

As we approach the final week of our diabetes management, we may begin looking back on the journey and wondering what has changed. Where has this path gotten us? The truth is, five weeks is a beginning, but we may already be able to see the fruits of wellness. As we continue, even after this six-week journey has been completed, we will realize that the fruit of the journey is life. When we embark on the road to diabetes management and wellness, we are more able to participate in the fullness of life.

### Faith Life
Today look back on your progress. Meditate for a few minutes, remembering where you started. Where have you found God on this journey?

### Medical
If you forget to take your medication for one dose, do not take a double dose. If you are not sure, call your primary care provider or pharmacist and ask whether you should take a dose immediately or wait until it is time for the next dose to get back on track.

## Movement
Today step up your aerobic exercise by quickening your pace or jogging intermittently. For example, walk for 10 minutes and then jog for 2.

## Work
How has this journey impacted your work life thus far? Have you noticed changes in your attitude, your work ethic, your productivity? Consider how you have changed your work life today and take note of your improvements.

## Emotional
Today keep a list of the different emotions that you feel throughout the day. If you notice a lot of "stressful" feelings, do some meditating or take a bath at the end of the day.

## Family and Friends
What do celebrations with your family and friends look like? Lots of sugary, fatty foods? Today write out a plan for the next celebration that you host. Include healthy foods and drinks.

## Nutrition
Instead of buying canned soups, try making a big pot of soup, either stove top or in a slow cooker. This way you can control the ingredients, and you can flavor the soup to your taste. Freeze the portions that you do not eat right away.

## Evening Wrap-up

*Or don't you know that all of us who were baptized
into Christ Jesus were baptized into his death?
We were therefore buried with him through
baptism into death in order that, just as Christ
was raised from the dead through the glory
of the Father, we too may live a new life.
For if we have been united with him in
a death like his, we will certainly also be
united with him in a resurrection like his.*
ROMANS 6:3–5

Our journey toward wellness and diabetes management is about abundant life. Abundant living might
mean something different to each of us, but we can
all agree that one of the fruits of wellness is abundant life. In Christian communities, we often talk
about being born again or receiving new life. On
this journey to diabetes management, we have the
opportunity to embrace a new life, which at times
can be like being born again.

*Most giving Lord, You have promised us life in abundance.
I pray today that You would help me embrace the
fruits of wellness. In Your holy name, Amen.*

# Day 35:
# Healing

## Morning Reflection

In many ways, this journey is about healing. It is about physical, spiritual, and emotional healing. Many of us have tried to feel better in the past. Maybe this six-week journey was a last resort found in a moment of desperation. The reality is, though, that the journey to diabetes management and wellness is a part of the healing process. We each experience healing in different ways. So today we will turn our focus to ways that we experience healing on this journey.

### Faith Life
Have you ever been healed? Keep in mind that healing can happen in many forms. Today take five minutes and write about what you think it means to be healed.

### Medical
If you have a fast-paced lifestyle, particularly one with an unpredictable schedule, ask your doctor about fast-acting insulin. This insulin can be taken just before eating and can help control your blood sugar within about thirty minutes.

## Movement
Exercise is incredibly healing. Today spend ten minutes warming up your muscles with some jumping jacks or jogging in place. Then spend at least five minutes stretching your muscles.

## Work
Do you ever go out for lunch as a part of your work? When you do, make sure to order a lower-sodium option, such as fish or a salad without cheese.

## Emotional
Physical healing means very little without emotional healing. Take ten minutes and write about a time in your life when you experienced emotional healing, such as a time when you have forgiven or been forgiven.

## Family and Friends
A large part of any healing is our support system. Today have a conversation with the members of your family and friends who are an important part of your support system. Tell them what healing on this journey looks like for you.

## Nutrition
Cheese is the number-one source of saturated fat in the American diet. It is also fairly high in sodium and cholesterol. Instead of adding cheese to your dishes today, try adding flavor with some lemon zest or a little vinegar.

## Evening Wrap-up

*Simon's mother-in-law was in bed with a fever,*
*and they immediately told Jesus about her.*
*So he went to her, took her hand and helped*
*her up. The fever left her and she began to wait*
*on them. That evening after sunset the people*
*brought to Jesus all the sick and demon-possessed.*
*The whole town gathered at the door, and Jesus*
*healed many who had various diseases.*
MARK 1:30–34

When we set out on this journey, many of us were tired, sick, frustrated, and in desperate need of some kind of healing in our lives. Now, on day thirty-five of this journey, we can see the healing that has happened so far. As we continue to move forward, we can experience healing in our lives. God offers us life in abundance, and as we strive for diabetes management and wellness, we can experience healing and fullness of life.

*Loving God, thank You for being a healing God.*
*Help me find healing on this journey toward wellness*
*and diabetes management. In Your holy name, Amen.*

# Week 6

## Tom's Story

When Tom's wife died ten years ago, he stopped taking care of himself. He ordered pizza several times a week. He stayed inside watching television most evenings. His doctor told him many times that he really needed to take better care of himself, but he continually put it off. "I just couldn't get out," Tom says.

But Tom's brother saw how unhealthy Tom was getting. He was gaining weight, he had diabetes, he was looking unwell. And so Tom's brother convinced him to join the Church Health Center. They began going to classes together. Tom learned how to cook for the first time in his life, and he began to exercise regularly.

When asked about his journey, Tom says that his brother's encouragement was the thing that changed his life. "He helped me to get up and go exercise, even when I didn't want to," Tom says.

Today Tom has lost about forty pounds and is feeling much better. He even disconnected his cable! Instead of watching television, he likes to go for a walk or cook a delicious meal. His diabetes is under control. He and his brother love to go on fishing trips together. "I am finally living again, praise God."

# Day 36:
## Conversion Stories

## Morning Reflection

Congratulations! We have reached the final weeks of our journey together. We have reached the end of this particular road. At this point in the journey, it can be helpful to figure out how to tell our stories. The journey to diabetes management and wellness is a path of conversion and growth. As we progress, learning how to tell our stories can help us to see both where we've been and where we want to go.

### Faith Life
Today spend five minutes writing about your wellness story. Was it gradual or sudden? What do you feel changed in your life?

### Medical
At this point in the journey, you may want to increase your exercise level. If you are going to engage in any kind of a rigorous exercise program, make sure that you talk to your doctor first. He or she can help you safely exercise.

### Movement
By now it would be a good idea to step up your exercise routine. Go for a slightly longer walk, using

weights, and do ten jumping jacks when you return. Do not forget to drink water and stretch!

## Work
During a break, grab a couple of coworkers and take a walk. Walk around your office, around the block, or go to a mall and walk for a while. Just give yourself a little activity and company to break up your day.

## Emotional
Many times quick conversions are what we could call mountaintop experiences. But the real work is done in the valleys. Today write about times that you have been on the mountaintop, and how those experiences translate to the work in the valleys.

## Family and Friends
Sometimes conversions can feel very lonely. Today go out and have fun with some friends or family members. They will help remind you that you are not alone.

## Nutrition
Canned vegetables and fruits can be easy and fast alternatives to fresh produce. However, they often come packaged in a good deal of salt and/or sugar. If you decide to use canned vegetables, use vegetables labeled "low sodium" and rinse them before you prepare them.

# Evening Wrap-up

*As he neared Damascus on his journey,*
*suddenly a light from heaven flashed around him.*
*He fell to the ground and heard a voice say to him,*
*"Saul, Saul, why do you persecute me?"*
*"Who are you, Lord?" Saul asked. "I am Jesus,*
*whom you are persecuting," he replied.*
*"Now get up and go into the city, and*
*you will be told what you must do."*
ACTS 9:3–6

On our journey to wellness and diabetes management, we have had mountaintop experiences and
life-changing moments. We know from Paul's experience that these conversions can happen very quickly.
But for most of us, those mountaintop experiences
are few and far between, and the real changes happen in the valleys. Even Paul, after he fell from his
horse and met Jesus, had to continue his life in the
valleys.

*God, in the mountains and valleys*
*You give me many opportunities for growth and change.*
*I pray today that You would help me embrace*
*my conversions as they come—whether they are on the*
*mountaintop or in the valley. In Your holy name, Amen.*

# Day 37:
## Knowing Ourselves

## Morning Reflection

In many ways this journey toward wellness and diabetes management can leave us unable to recognize ourselves from the person we were when we began. And so now at the end of our six-week journey, we have a need to look at ourselves and get to know who we are again. We can take a step back from the journey itself to reflect on who we are becoming and who we used to be.

### Faith Life
What does it mean to love yourself? Spend five minutes writing about loving yourself. Keep in mind that God loves you and has commanded you to love your neighbor as yourself. This means that you must love your neighbor and yourself.

### Medical
Talk to your care provider about the amount of alcohol you can safely consume. Most medical experts recommend no more than two alcoholic beverages a day for men, and no more than one for women. Remember that alcohol consumption can affect your glucose levels.

## Movement
Today as you cook dinner or wait for a phone call, do three sets of ten wall push-ups. Try to lower yourself a little deeper with each push-up. You should feel your heart rate increase slightly and the muscles in your arms and abdominals working.

## Work
If you must go out for lunch at work, try to avoid eating fast food. Instead try to find a place where you can order lean protein and vegetables that are not fried.

## Emotional
At the end of the day today, find some time to care for yourself, whatever that means. Take a bath, read a book, call some friends to hang out. Relieving stress and caring for yourself is a crucial element to managing diabetes.

## Family and Friends
When you plan activities with your family and friends, try going to a park, playground, or museum instead of going immediately to a restaurant. This way you will have some kind of physical activity built into your outing. Many cities have "free days" at museums for a low-cost activity.

## Nutrition
Sodium, saturated fat, sugar, and cholesterol can be hidden in foods that otherwise look healthy. Do not count on pictures or names for nutrition information. Remember, read the food label before you buy!

## Evening Wrap-up

*You have searched me, L*ORD*, and you know me.*
*You know when I sit and when I rise;*
*you perceive my thoughts from afar.*
*You discern my going out and my lying down;*
*you are familiar with all my ways. . . .*
*For you created my inmost being; you knit me*
*together in my mother's womb. I praise you*
*because I am fearfully and wonderfully made;*
*your works are wonderful, I know that full well."*
PSALM 139:1–3, 13–14

We are on this journey toward wellness, and each of us has experienced change and transformation, even in places where we least expected it. But we can take solace in the fact that God knows us intimately. God has created our innermost being, and God remains constant even as we feel everything is changing. On this journey toward diabetes management, God continues to know us, even when we feel we do not know ourselves.

*Loving God, I know that I am fearfully and wonderfully*
*made. Help me to embrace the changes*
*in myself and to rely on Your constancy.*
*In Your holy name, Amen.*

# Day 38:
## The Next Steps

## Morning Reflection

Now at the end of our journey, it is time to look forward past our six weeks together and into the next phase of the journey. As we have said all along, the journey to wellness and diabetes management is a lifelong process. When we began, we identified "first steps" that we needed to take. Now at the end, we can identify those next steps that will allow us to move forward from here.

### Faith Life
Today take five minutes and reflect on how far you've come in this journey. Then turn your focus to the future.

### Medical
Understand that diabetes can come with a host of complications, such as hypertension and high cholesterol. During your next doctor's visit, ask about what your numbers are.

### Movement
Try to begin incorporating movement into your day-to-day mundane activities. For example, if you run to the store to buy a gallon of milk, carry the milk with you instead of putting it in a cart. Then

while you stand in line, do some alternating bicep curls with it.

## Work
Bring an insulated lunch bag to work with some raw chopped vegetables such as celery, carrots, and red bell peppers to snack on when you get hungry. If you want to add a little spice, throw in a few radishes as well.

## Emotional
Moving forward from here may be intimidating. Today make a list of stress-relieving activities that you have learned over the past six weeks.

## Family and Friends
Your family and friends will be very important to your journey. Today try to set up a regular walking time with one or more of your friends or family members. Having a regular time will help you to get into (and stay in) the habit of walking.

## Nutrition
Aim for five servings of vegetables in a day. To get all of those servings, try serving at least two different vegetables with dinner. Tonight try a cooked option (like steamed broccoli) and a raw option (such as some sliced red peppers or a salad).

## Evening Wrap-up

*Let us draw near to God with a sincere heart and with the full assurance that faith brings, having our hearts sprinkled to cleanse us from a guilty conscience and having our bodies washed with pure water. Let us hold unswervingly to the hope we profess, for he who promised is faithful. And let us consider how we may spur one another on toward love and good deeds, not giving up meeting together, as some are in the habit of doing, but encouraging one another—and all the more as you see the Day approaching.*
HEBREWS 10:22–25

The journey toward wellness and diabetes management, and it is about hope. As we move forward beyond this six-week journey, we can hold on to the hope that we have, knowing that God is faithful and walks with us.

*Faithful God, help me today to hold on to the hope that I have placed in You. Continue to walk with me even as I step beyond this six-week journey into the rest of my life. In Your holy name, Amen.*

# Day 39:
# Fellow Travelers

## Morning Reflection

This is not a journey that we can undertake alone. We have a team of health-care professionals who help us on the journey, but we also have friends, family, and other fellow travelers who can walk the journey with us. As we move forward, we must learn how to rely on others who can encourage us when we need it and who can celebrate with us when we succeed.

### Faith Life

Does your faith community have Sunday school programs? Today consider starting up a Sunday school program that is centered on the wellness journey. Encourage other members of your faith community to live wellness-oriented lives.

### Medical

Remember that medication is not a magical pill. When your physician writes a prescription for a medication, ask questions about what lifestyle changes you should be making along with the medication to be healthier.

## Movement

Today before your family sits down for dinner, go for a walk together. Doing some exercise before you eat will make you feel better and will give you a better gauge on your appetite.

## Work

If there is someone at your work who shares your particular lunchtime, and perhaps is interested in eating healthy meals, adopt that person as a lunch buddy. Take turns bringing in new, healthy dishes to try.

## Emotional

When we feel alone, we can become despondent, and it can really halt our progress on the wellness journey. Today spend five minutes writing about the many ways in which you are not alone.

## Family and Friends

Your family and friends can be a great support, but it can also be good to seek support from people who are going through a similar experience to yours. Support groups exist at gyms and wellness centers as well as online. Find a group that you can belong to.

## Nutrition

No matter how much you want to lose weight, do not start a fad diet. While they may help you lose weight, fad diets generally do not promote overall wellness, as they often include unbalanced meal plans.

## Evening Wrap-up

*"My command is this: Love each other as I have
loved you. Greater love has no one than this:
to lay down one's life for one's friends.
You are my friends if you do what I command. . . .
You did not choose me, but I chose you and
appointed you so that you might go and bear
fruit—fruit that will last—and so that whatever
you ask in my name the Father will give you."*
JOHN 15:12–14, 16

As we continue on this journey, we will need to find
fellow travelers who can encourage us on the way.
We have friends, family, and acquaintances who
can encourage us, as well as health professionals
who certainly care for us. But we are reminded in
this passage from John that the fellow traveler who
is most consistently with us is Jesus. Christ is the
one who walks the journey to wellness with us.

*Loving God, You have walked with me on this journey.
I pray that You would continue to travel with me,
wherever I find myself. In Your holy name, Amen.*

# Day 40:
## Forty Days

## Morning Reflection

Today is day forty—congratulations! You have made it forty days! Over the past six weeks you have gained the skills necessary to continue on your journey toward diabetes management. Setbacks will probably happen from time to time, but you have set up a foundation that you can return to when needed. The journey to diabetes management may take you to unexpected places, but wherever wellness takes you, it is sure to lead to a fuller and more abundant life.

### Faith Life

At the end of this six-week journey, we can begin to imagine life beyond this series. In particular we can think about abundant living, which after all, has been the goal. Take five minutes today and write about what you think abundant living means in your life now.

### Medical

If you change health-care providers, try to get to know them while you are healthy. It is much easier for doctors to treat you when they know what "healthy you" is like.

## Movement
In celebration of reaching the fortieth day of managing diabetes, put on some music and dance around your house. Laugh as you want to, and let go of your inhibitions for a while.

## Work
If you need to go out to lunch for work, order water instead of calorie- or caffeine-laden drinks. Replacing sugary drinks with water—over the long haul—will make a difference. Add lemon for taste. Your taste buds will adjust to this new flavor, and soon you may find that you crave water!

## Emotional
Today try to rest. When we are tired, overworked, and sleep deprived, our bodies respond to stressors, causing us to hang on to weight, which can contribute to diabetes.

## Family and Friends
Today prepare a meal for your friends and family that you have never prepared before. Get your guests to help you prepare the meal, chopping vegetables or stirring the pot as things cook.

## Nutrition
When you go out to eat, ask for a to-go container to come with your food. When your food comes, put half your meal in the to-go container to prevent overeating.

## Evening Wrap-up

*"Arise, shine, for your light has come,*
*and the glory of the LORD rises upon you.*
*See, darkness covers the earth and thick darkness*
*is over the peoples, but the LORD rises upon you*
*and his glory appears over you. Nations will come*
*to your light, and kings to the brightness of your*
*dawn. . . . Then you will look and be radiant,*
*your heart will throb and swell with joy."*
ISAIAH 60:1–3, 5

Remember that God gives us abundant grace through Jesus Christ and that we are not only given abundant grace in spirit, but in our whole selves and our whole lives. This journey to wellness is about responding appropriately to that abundant grace that Jesus Christ grants us. When we care for ourselves, we are caring for God's creation—the very thing that Jesus came to save.

*Loving God, You have offered me an abundant and full life.*
*You have blessed me in countless ways.*
*I pray that You would continue to walk with me*
*as I find ways to embrace the abundant living that*
*You have offered me. In Your holy name, Amen.*

# Day 41:
## Review

---

## Morning Reflection

Now that the forty days are over, today will be a day of review. When we started this journey, we had to assess where we were in order to set goals for the future. In a similar manner, we have to assess where we are again, so that we can know where we need to go from here. We need to see our successes as well as our setbacks, so that we recognize the things we still need to work on.

### Faith Life

When we started, you wrote ten words describing your faith life. Again take five minutes and write ten words describing your faith life now. Compare the two lists. What has changed? What has stayed the same?

### Medical

Has your medical situation changed? Take a few minutes today and look at how far you have come in the last six weeks.

### Movement

Go for a walk today and walk as far as you can walk. How far could you walk the first time you did this? Can you feel the improvement in the way your body is reacting to the exercise?

### Work
What has changed about your work environment? Are you drinking more water? Are you eating healthier snacks? Are you getting a little exercise throughout the day?

### Emotional
What has changed in your emotional wellness? Take a look at your emotional highs and lows from week two. Do you still have similar highs and lows, or has your overall emotional pattern changed a bit?

### Family and Friends
What have your family and friends thought about your journey? Can they see a difference in you? Take a moment today and ask one or two of them.

### Nutrition
In the first week, you made a list of the foods that you like to eat. Can you expand that list any after six weeks? In particular, can you include more healthy meals on that list?

# Evening Wrap-up

*I have fought the good fight,*
*I have finished the race,*
*I have kept the faith.*
2 TIMOTHY 4:7

The last six weeks have been challenging in a variety of ways. You have been asked to try vastly new things, from food to exercises. You have been asked to step outside of your comfort zone, to explore emotions that most of us do not take the time to explore regularly. But the journey—at least this part of the journey—is finished. And you have finished the race. For that, you ought to be very proud and thankful. You have run the race, and God has been running right beside you. Remember as you continue from this point, God runs the race with you. God gives us all strength and endurance when we most need it, and God cheers when we cross the finish line.

*God of all things, thank You for the gift of wellness.*
*Help me continue on this journey with endurance*
*and bravery. In Your holy name, Amen.*

# Day 42:
## Looking Ahead

## Morning Reflection

With the six weeks completed, it can certainly feel like the journey is over. However as we have said before, the journey has really only just begun. The journey to wellness is never over. Life will offer us many surprises along the way, and it will be part of the journey to adapt as life happens. Today as we close this chapter, we look ahead to continue the lessons learned on this road.

### Faith Life
As you continue on this journey, remember to take time to pray or meditate each day. Prayer and meditation can keep you connected to your purpose and your anchor.

### Medical
Take all medication exactly as prescribed, and do not be afraid to talk to your doctor about anything. The best way to stay medically healthy is to have open communication with your physician.

### Movement
Move everywhere. Find ways to add a few steps to your day in everything that you do. A great goal would be to add two hundred steps one day, four

hundred the next day, and keep adding two hundred steps each day throughout the week. This will help your body to burn calories more efficiently each day.

## Work
Try to find time in your days to exercise even a little bit. It will help break up the monotony of the day and will help you add a few steps. Also avoid office junk food. Instead opt for healthy snacks and lunches.

## Emotional
Find and remember ways that you can relieve stress. Take a hot bath, go for a walk, read a book. Just find something that works for you and do it every day. The more you relieve your stress, the better you will feel, and the healthier you will become.

## Family and Friends
Remember that your family and friends are your support system. When you are struggling, do not be afraid to lean on them for support, and when you have succeeded, do not be afraid to celebrate with them.

## Nutrition
Make your calories count. Enjoy all the wonderful colors and flavors of God's creation as you prepare meals using whole grains, a variety of fruits and vegetables, and lean meats—but let yourself splurge on occasion!

## Evening Wrap-up

*Finally, brothers and sisters, whatever is true,*
*whatever is noble, whatever is right,*
*whatever is pure, whatever is lovely,*
*whatever is admirable—if anything is excellent*
*or praiseworthy—think about such things.*
*Whatever you have learned or received or heard*
*from me, or seen in me—put it into practice.*
*And the God of peace will be with you.*
PHILIPPIANS 4:8–9

It has been a long journey to this point, but you have been given many tools to continue. You will find other tools to add to your toolbox, and you will have setbacks. But remember that God walks with you, and God can grant you peace, even when you have a difficult time finding it for yourself.

*God of peace, be with me as I continue on this journey.*
*Help me remember the things I have learned, and help me*
*continue learning. I will continue to strive to honor*
*my body and my whole self, Your creation.*
*In Your holy name, Amen.*

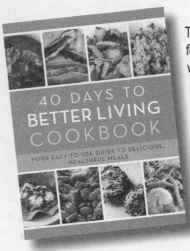